I0090189

Intermittent Fasting for Women
30-Day Challenge

Complete Weight Loss Guide for Women: Burn Fat, Slim Down, and Heal Your Body

By Susan Katz

© Copyright 2018 - All rights reserved.

The content contained within this book may not be reproduced, duplicated or transmitted without direct written permission from the author or the publisher.

Under no circumstances will any blame or legal responsibility be held against the publisher, or author, for any damages, reparation, or monetary loss due to the information contained within this book. Either directly or indirectly.

Legal Notice:

This book is copyright protected. This book is only for personal use. You cannot amend, distribute, sell, use, quote or paraphrase any part, or the content within this book, without the consent of the author or publisher.

Disclaimer Notice:

Please note the information contained within this document is for educational and entertainment purposes only. All effort has been executed to present accurate, up to date, and reliable, complete information. No warranties of any kind are declared or implied. Readers acknowledge that the author is not engaging in the rendering of legal, financial, medical or professional advice. The content within this book has been derived from various sources. Please consult a licensed professional before attempting any techniques outlined in this book.

By reading this document, the reader agrees that under no circumstances is the author responsible for any losses, direct or indirect, which are incurred as a result of the use of the information contained within this document, including, but not limited to, — errors, omissions, or inaccuracies.

Table of Contents

Introduction

Imagine this: you are on a beach in Miami, wearing your floral wrap-around dress and a two-piece swimsuit underneath. You feel confident as ever; the wind in your face, the warm water splashes on your legs. It feels so real to finally feel sexy. You feel like everybody has been staring at you the whole time but not in a negative way. It merely feels as if they are in awe of your beauty and body. You feel young and beautiful; it is like you can conquer the world once again with your profound body.

This time, you remember what it feels to be a bullied teenager in high school. Think of the names that the bullies used to yell at you over and over again. Whale! Pig! Ugly! It does not seem to add much, but it hurts more than they know. People saw you as a source of traffic – a nuisance in society - because of your weight. I mean, you cannot ride the bus without experiencing the judging stares, telling you that your body covers two seats and that it is better if you stand up for the benefit of others than to remain sitting.

Sometimes, you feel embarrassed to ask for an extra scoop of ice cream or an extra bowl of salad without the customers' and waiters' eyes trained on you as well. It feels so sad to live the life of an overweight teenager. It seems like every day is a trial that you outwait until you get home and rest, only to repeat the same cycle the next day.

There are many reasons why a woman grows stout. One of them is aging. But this should not make you stop striving to have the sexy body that you deserve. Imagine still getting to wear your two-piece at the age of 40. People would ask, "How old are you?" They would not believe their eyes even when you tell them that you are already 45 years old. With the body of a superstar, you will be mistaken as someone in your early 20s. Trust me when I say that you can still regain that super-hot body of yours.

Giving birth is the most magical event of all time. However, it has a lot of physical effects on the mother, especially without exercise and proper diet. Most moms let themselves go and give no regard to their bodies after birth. But sooner than later, they start to regret the extra pounds that they have gained from being a full-time mother. If you are having the same problems, you have come to the right place. Who said you cannot be sexy again in a matter of 30 days? YOU CAN, AND YOU WILL! Let me guide you through it step by step.

If you are afraid that people will judge you by having this book, don't be! There are millions of women out there who would give anything to be led on the road to weight loss by hand. Better yet, be proud that you are doing something for yourself to achieve a goal and feel young, beautiful, and sexy from the inside and out.

The History of Fasting and Weight Loss

Our ancestors have started fasting as early as the 3rd century BC when the Greeks regarded stoutness as a form of physical abnormality – a result of corruption, sloth, and greed. This was the reason why their scientists such as Hippocrates recommended the balance between extremities, introducing a smooth and sensible lifestyle that could help the people get back in shape. Hippocrates, being the father of medicine, focused his energy and research in highlighting the importance of understanding the health of the patient, the independence and health of mind, the harmony deep within the individual, and the social and natural environments he lives in. He constituted the saying that goes, "A healthy mind in a healthy body", which is one of the main principles of the Hippocratic philosophy. He was the first person to believe that diseases were not brought at all by demons and spirits. Rather, they were brought by either physical deprivation or gluttony. He also found that people can cope with these illnesses through a balanced diet, rest, and healthy physical activities.

It was Hippocrates who proposed the relationship between the body and the mind. An ill body could cause an ill mind, and vice versa. He claimed in his research that a person's beliefs, ideas, thought, and feelings, came from the brain, not the heart, and it had a significant effect to the physiological aspect of a person. Obviously so, whenever we are depressed, we are less inclined to work and concentrate. We feel as if every part of our body hurts as much as our heart. But if we feel happy, we are more energetic and motivated to get things done and go through a whole day no matter how hard it is. This theory of the Father of Medicine can be quite useful in our journey towards weight loss. Nevertheless, we will get more into that later.

In a more specific sense, fasting has its own roots that dates back to Hippocrates as well. Over the years, the method has been a time-tested tradition. It is not only used for weight loss but also for improving concentration, extending human life, preventing Alzheimer's disease, increasing insulin resistance, and even slowing down the aging process. The theory of fasting comes from the idea that lowering the insulin levels promote weight gain. The problem is that all foods significantly increase the levels of insulin in the body. So, the only way to lose weight effectively is to abstain from food. Hence, the term 'fasting' was born.

According to experts, one of the most common mistakes done by people who try to lose weight is searching for an all-exotic food variety that can make them lose weight. Others resort to products that are meant for slimming, which they do not know are harmful to the body and might cause more trouble than good when taken. Some specialists have come up with the conclusion that the only way to significantly feel weight loss is through old and proven methods like fasting.

You would be surprised to know who initiated the revolution towards fasting. After all, it was no other than Hippocrates of Cos. He was the one who started the consumption of apple cider vinegar to lose weight. According to one of his principles, "To eat when you are sick is to feed your illness." This was later echoed by the Greek writer and historian named Plutarch who claimed, "Instead of using a medicine, better fast today." Other researchers claimed that even Plato and his student Aristotle were both advocates of the concept of fasting. Scientists from ancient Greece believed that this method was known as the "physician within." It is the instinct that makes not only humans but also animals anorexic when they get sick. This can be observed in modern times when there is a significant decline in appetite whenever a person is ill. Apparently, there is an internal rationale for feeling that way, and it should not be ignored. Most of us are forced to take in chunks of food even when we have no appetite. Our doctors and parents would urge us to eat a significant amount of food when we get sick. "Eat your food so that you can take your medicine" - this is the most common sentence we hear whenever we acquire an illness. However, what if we start to listen to our forefathers and believe we merely feed the virus in our body when we eat? Or, even if we do, we should resort to healthy foods and count the calories much like what Lulu Peters and William Banting had proposed. Our bodies have their own antibacterial properties. Can't you see that the main reason why viruses and bacteria get stronger every day is because of the countless breakthroughs and innovation in medicine?

Let us take a look at the opinions of other intellectual giants. The founder of toxicology, Philip Paracelsus, was also a great supporter of fasting. He is one of the three founders of modern Western medicine along with Hippocrates and Galen, who wrote that fasting is the greatest remedy. This idea was supported by Benjamin Franklin, one of America's founding fathers, who said that the best of all medicines is resting and fasting. In a religious perspective, did you know that Jesus Christ, Buddha, and Muhammed shared the same belief regarding the benefits of fasting? According to their wisdom, the practice aids in cleansing and purification the body. In Buddhism, food is only consumed in the morning, and the followers do not eat anything for the rest of the day. Hence, the first meal in the morning is known as breakfast. Meaning, "to break the fasting." For Muslims, it is an important part of tradition to fast from sunrise to sunset during Ramadan, their holy month. The Prophet Muhammad encouraged people to skip meals on Mondays and Thursdays every week as well. As you can see, fasting indeed withstood the hands of time. Until now, it is recognized as one of the most effective ways to stay healthy.

However, whenever some individuals think about the process of fasting, they become skeptic towards its effects on the human body. Other assume that the practice means starvation and self-torture. To set things straight, fasting is way too different from starvation. First and foremost, when you say the latter, it entails an involuntary absence of food, which is often the effect of poverty or lack of resources. The former term, meanwhile, refers to voluntary abstinence for physical, spiritual, and mental purposes. When you fast, you choose when and what to eat. These two words should not be mistaken with each other because they are not the same. One of the main reasons why I am writing this book is to enlighten people about the advantages of fasting and to break the stigma that many have associated with this golden process.

Types of Fasting

There are several fasting methods out there. Although some of them might not be as famous as intermittent fasting, it is best to have an idea about the others for the sake of having choices in the long run. Who knows, maybe after you have successfully reached your ideal body structure, you can try other practices and discover more than what meets the eye.

Occasional Short Fasts

This type of fasting is the starting point for most people. This does not follow a consistent schedule; it merely constitutes an occasional fast for six, 12 or 24 hours. There is not much commitment to this technique, though, there is no guarantee that it will work. See, some people indeed engage in fasting. The problem is, when it is time for them to eat, they consume food voraciously, forgetting what they have just done before that and why.

Intermittent Fasting

Intermittent fasting, as mentioned earlier, is one of the

most effective ways of fasting because it requires commitment and a whole new level of discipline. This method is defined as a regular act of abstinence. For example, you skip meals for one, two or three days a week. In the succeeding chapters, we will be discussing the power and practices related to intermittent fasting. From what some experts have said, after all, it is a form of partial fasting that helps you develop a dietary routine. Apart from the fact that it helps you control your eating habits, it can also allow you to do other activities, such as sports and hobbies.

Longer Fasts

This is by one of the most difficult kinds of fasting because it entails that you will abstain from eating for three days to one week. It is far more difficult than intermittent fasting and requires times ten of commitment and discipline. Plus, most people who start fasting with this technique end up giving up because they cannot endure the hunger, pain, and discomfort that come with longer fasts.

Extended Fasting

Extended fasting is another challenging form of fasting since it means that you will extend a scheduled fast for two hours or more. Imagine going beyond a three-day fast. Imagine the discipline and self-control needed for such ordeal. Much like longer fasts, you need to have an experience with this method already and be able to master your thoughts. Otherwise, you might be doing more harm than good to your body.

Open-Ended Fasts

An open-ended fast is one of the most common fasting techniques of all time. When you do it, you can break your commitment to the method after reaching your goals. Extended fasts and intermittent fasting are a couple of its examples. Then, you may resort to occasional fasting to maintain your health and physical appearance.

Occasional or Longer Group Fasting

There are organizations that facilitate occasional group

fasting. This can help you stay on track towards a successful fast. There is a leader to monitor your achievements every day, every week, and every month. Whenever you feel sad or down about not being able to live life to the fullest, you can open up to your superiors to gain uplifting advices to get you to keep on fasting.

Chapter 1: Intermittent Fasting for Women

If you are looking for the best way to lose weight in just 30 days, you have come to the right place! In this book, I am not only teaching you how to fast intermittently, but I am also incorporating some methods of motivation and self-discipline. As our father of medicine, Hippocrates, has theorized, there is a back-and-forth connection between the body and mind. Without a proper mindset, intermittent fasting will not be as effective as you want it to be, regardless of how long you do it.

The answer to your prayers does not lie on the new diets that you see on the web. You cannot depend on the dietary supplements in the stores either. You see, even if you try it all, nothing can make you lose weight if you have no idea about the power of fasting. Furthermore, none of those methods have withstood the test of time as much as fasting has. Even when you adopt one of the most famous weight-loss methods out there, how sure are you that you will not develop any illness in the future because of it? How can you tell with certainty that you will not revert to your old body once you stop following the fad?

Of course, to sell their products, the creators of new diets and dietary supplements will claim that they are "guaranteed safe and effective." However, after 10 or 20 years of usage, who can ensure that you will not contract a chronic disease due to the chemicals and substances that are in such products?

The so-called "treatments" mentioned above have not been proven effective in a matter of centuries. The people who have employed fasting as a method of weight loss, on the other hand, have reported to be more alert and energetic in their daily activities. Several celebrities do intermittent fasting as well to maintain their bodies and maintain a healthy lifestyle. Some of the female personalities who do so include Beyoncé, Jennifer Lopez, Selena Gomez, Nicole Kidman, and Miranda Kerr. For the men, we have Benedict Cumberbatch, Hugh Jackman, Terry Crews, and Chris

Hemsworth. If you are wondering how they get the energy to accomplish all of their activities in Hollywood, it must have something to do with fasting intermittently.

Other famous people such as Kourtney Kardashian, Moby, Molly Sims, Chris Pratt, and Paul Krugman also swear to intermittent fasting. John Kane, who experimented on the practice, claimed that ever since he started employing the method, he had been brighter, sharper, and happier than ever in life. He said that it could wake people up and hype up the energy. Although he did not follow any standard plan of fasting, he benefited from it and was contented with the results.

As easy as it may seem not to eat, some individuals cannot stick to intermittent fasting. The main reason is lack of discipline and motivation. For people who have been used to a voracious lifestyle, after all, it is hard for them to say no when they see a muffin, cake, junk food, or other enticing stuff in the corner or the ref. Because of their frustration, they get stressed out, depressed, anxious, and apprehended, causing them to binge-eat and gain weight even more. The problem with these individuals is not their food intake. Instead, it is their mindset towards the methods of weight loss. This is the main reason why we need to discuss several ways to train your mind before fasting in the following chapters.

Intermittent Fasting

The popularity of intermittent fasting among countries is spreading like a wildfire in this era. From the term itself, intermittent fasting (IF) is a pattern of eating and not eating during a specific period. The process involves limiting your caloric intake in certain days or weeks by merely allowing you to consume foods in a few hours daily. For example, you may eat breakfast, but you cannot any food for the rest of the day. Others employ time as their signal to eat. Some people only eat at 7 in the morning and in the evening without consuming anything in between.

Though its main cause of fame is its relation to weight loss, intermittent fasting was first used for disease prevention and longevity. Its ability to help you lose weight is just a bonus. Studies have shown that when food is restricted from lab rats and other species such as mice, hamsters, and yeast, this can extend their lifespan by a significant amount of time. As mentioned earlier, this procedure has also supported the theory of Paracelsus and Hippocrates when they advise people not to eat when they are sick. Modern research has found that bad cells are being killed in the process of fasting, too, so it seems to enhance the body's ability to counteract foreign bodies.

In the year 2017, researchers have worked together to know whether fasting can reduce the onset of diabetes, cancer, and cardiovascular diseases. In this study, they have randomized 100 samples into two groups for three months. The first group was allowed to eat anything they want, and the latter group fasted for days each month. After the experimentation, the researchers have gathered that fasting can really improve someone's health. It caused weight loss, lowered blood pressure, and decreased the genetic marker for cancer, the IGF–1. However, there were a lot of people who gave up in the fasting phase, which led them to believe that fasting is a difficult but effective method. Apart from this conclusion, though, there are other surprising benefits of intermittent fasting to human beings.

If you aim to reach your maximum height potential, consider fasting as a way to boost your human growth hormone (HGH). The practice makes it skyrocket in your body and allows you to grow taller and leaner as time goes by. The levels of insulin can also normalize through fasting by making stored body fat more accessible for expending or burning. Researches have also found that intermittent fasting can contribute to cellular repair - a process that gets rid of dead cells and dysfunctional proteins that build up inside human cells. It can also increase your metabolic rate by 3.6% to 14%, thus deeming it the most powerful tool for weight loss. In a study conducted in 2016, people who employed intermittent fasting as a weight-loss remedy showed a significant rate of 3% to 8% weight reduction in 3 -24 weeks' time. The same researchers also gathered that people could reduce their waistline by 4% to 7% through intermittent fasting.

In a more serious note, intermittent fasting also prevents

inflammation in the body, which is the key indicator of chronic diseases. Hippocrates and John Kane were right by saying that this method could improve your alertness and energy. Furthermore, studies show that the practice does not only make you lose weight but also promote brain health and prevent Alzheimer's disease. Other researchers have revealed that intermittent fasting can detoxify the body. It helps you get rid of harmful chemicals and substances that may cause diseases. In turn, it promotes cell regeneration as early as 2-4 days since following the method. From the data gathered, intermittent fasting can aid in boosting the immune system as well, protecting the body and its cells from foreign entities, as well as cellular damage that's due to external factors like UV rays and chemotherapy.

Who Should Not Fast?

It is no secret that not all individuals are allowed to fast. People with eating disorders and depression, for instance, should not try fasting at all because it worsens their condition and might cause serious damages to the body. We have discussed at the beginning of the chapter how serotonin, being the happy hormone, works against depression. It is needed to avert the effects of sadness and frustration, and it can only be acquired through food intake. Depressed patients are required to eat three times a day with snacks in between to promote the secretion of serotonin, which usually comes from the breakdown of food into sugar. Without ample food in the body, the person stays depressed and may even start entertaining suicidal thoughts.

Anorexia nervosa patients should not be allowed to fast as well. This eating disorder is characterized by excessive weight loss or lack of sufficient weight gain. It inhibits an individual from maintaining an appropriate weight, height, and stature for a specific age. Moreover, people with anorexia nervosa have a distorted body image. They see themselves as overweight even when they no longer have any fat to burn, and they appear all skin and bones to normal folks. This disorder can affect all ages, though it usually starts in adolescence when people - especially women - seek a sense of belonging in groups. When a lady has anorexia, for instance, she will not eat and probably starve herself to look good in her own eyes. She tends to deny her hunger when others ask why she won't eat; even when she does pick up the fork and spoon, she will take an excessive amount of laxatives to expel the calories taken. If not, the lady might force herself to regurgitate all the food and exercise extraneously just to "get in shape." Anorexia nervosa is one of the scariest eating disorders because it can lead to severe conditions, such as stomach cancer, ulcer, and death. We have even gathered that the "anything goes" mentality that some experts permit during the feeding state can make someone overeat and create guilt, shame, and other problems that can only become worse over time. For someone with emotional or psychological eating disorders, intermittent fasting can, therefore, become a convenient crutch to amplify such issues.

Furthermore, fasting can be helpful for individuals dealing with gut issues, stress, and anxiety. When you have gastroesophageal reflux disorder (GERD), a form of a stomach illness, fasting is not recommended either. This illness is characterized by heartburn or acid indigestion since the stomach does not have enough food to churn.

The problem is, some experts say that fasting can amplify anxiety and stress in certain individuals. Apparently, once folks with these conditions fast, they tend to be "hangry" when there is an imbalance of cortisol in the body. They become temperamental, irritable, and anxious, thus leaving them either aggressive or unproductive throughout the day. If you notice such symptoms in yourself, consult your doctor or psychiatrist before you employ fasting as a weight-loss remedy.

Pregnant and breastfeeding mothers should not be allowed to fast as well. You will need every nutrient you can get to help your child develop in the womb. Also, when you are underweight and undernourished, you no longer need to fast. Instead, you need to do the opposite and eat as many foods as you can to compensate for your insufficient weight. When you are trying to conceive children, maintain a healthy diet, but avoid fasting. This can cause hormonal imbalance, which makes conception a more difficult process.

Having amenorrhea is also an indication for women that

fasting is not for you. This condition is characterized by the absence of menstruation for months at a time. When you have an irregular cycle, it is possible that you are not using enough subcutaneous fat as energy during menstruation. You may lack in nutrients needed for the blood to circulate properly in your body as well, thus throwing your hormones and bodily chemicals out of balance. One of the most common causes of amenorrhea is pregnancy. So, when you have a missed period, check for any signs of pregnancy and do not fast. Instead, consume many fruits, vegetables, and every nutritious food in the book, including water.

Also, when you are under medications for certain illnesses, such as diabetes and anemia, make sure that you have your physician's go signal before fasting. There are instances when medicines work poorly without the assistance of food to absorb the substances.

Disadvantages of Fasting

Much like any other weight-loss method, there are also disadvantages of intermittent fasting that we should not ignore. From the experiments and observations conducted by doctors, they have found that fasting can cause dehydration to people because the body does not get enough food. Fasting is also known to increase stress and disrupt sleep as it aids in the secretion of cortisol in the body. If you do not get enough food, you may become more irritable and agitated. It can cause headache, stomach ache, and muscle pain, especially during hard work. Nausea can also be a common effect of fasting because of the lack of sugar in the body. It is true the practice can lower blood pressure, too; however, excessive fasting can do that at a dangerous rate. Scientists and experts have also found that the method contributes to heartburn and acidity because of the unexpended stomach acids.

Myths about Intermittent Fasting

1.   It Is Dangerous to Your Health.

When people think about fasting, they roll their eyes and assume that it will be bad for your health. They will even dissuade you from doing it because these individuals believe that it can do more harm than good to you. What they do not understand is the effects and science of doing intermittent fasting as you go along. As long as you have been given permission to do so, I do not see why you cannot try it.

2. You Should Not Drink Liquids When Fasting.

This is one of the reasons why people remain skeptic about the powers of intermittent fasting. In reality, you can drink coffee, green tea, and water in between your fast breaks to avoid ulcer and other gut-related illnesses.

3. Skipping Breakfast Is Unhealthy.

There is a stigma that says people who skip breakfast have unhealthy lifestyles. Many folks fast for various reasons, not just to lose weight. Just look at the health benefits that intermittent fasting can bring to your body. If you choose a fasting schedule that requires you to skip breakfast, it should not be a problem. Others do that all the time even if they are not fasting. They prefer having a meal in between instead, which you might know more of as 'brunch.'

4.   You Cannot Take Supplements While Fasting.

Food supplements are excellent sources of vitamins and minerals that the body requires. When you are employing intermittent fasting as a means of living healthily, it is perfectly okay to take them while following the IF method.

5.   Fasting Can Cause Muscle Loss.

Every weight-loss method has this side effect, and intermittent fasting is not any different. Nevertheless, you can counter it by taking high levels of protein and maintaining regular exercise even when you are fasting to promote muscle building.

6.   Children Can Fast, Too.

Kids are not allowed to fast at all. Even if your child is obese or overweight, he or she should not be subjected to intermittent fasting. To help them lose weight, it is important to promote another technique, such as the fruit diet, water cleansing, regular exercise, and reduction of caloric intake in every meal.

Chapter 2: Science behind Intermittent Fasting

Hippocrates and his colleagues did not develop the concept of fasting by using their instinct or opinions. It took them years of experimentation, as well as observing individuals who experienced it. They even tried fasting themselves to see and feel its effects within the human body.

In this chapter, I will be discussing how fasting works. To be specific, how does the method affect the cells? What does it do to promote its health benefits? Understanding the science behind this concept is a vital tool to garner an idea on how it can useful for you. I am sure you do not want to be shocked by the sudden changes it can bring as you continue to fast intermittently. We have also discussed in the previous chapters that fasting is not for everyone. Knowing what it should feel like now can help you understand if it is right for you or not. You also need to know if you are doing it properly or not.

Every minute of every day, our body needs energy. Whether we are resting, procrastinating or engaging in strenuous work, we need sugar to kickstart our organs and keep our blood flowing efficiently in our veins. The form of sugar we need in our body to be converted into energy is called carbohydrates, which are found in grains, dairy products, fruits, vegetables, beans, concessionaires, and others. Our muscles and liver secrete glucose to our bloodstream, especially when the body is performing an activity. Without it, you can become weaker and might not be able to accomplish any task for the day.

When a person engages in fasting, this whole process changes. After about eight hours of food abstinence, the liver will have used up all its glucose reserves up to the last drop. When this happens, the body goes into a state called gluconeogenesis, which switches the body into fasting mode. In this phase, you increase the number of calories that you burn. Without the glucose secreted by the liver, it generates its own form of energy using the fats inside the body, thus promoting weight loss. However, fasting becomes starvation when there are no more fats to use up. This causes dangerous effects on the body; that's why you need to break this fast on a timely yet efficient schedule. Without any fat to burn, your metabolism starts to slow down, and you will start to burn muscles for energy, so your muscle mass will reduce and put the body in a more hazardous state.

Types of Intermittent Fasting

It is imperative to take fasting as more than a mere hobby. Without proper guidance and schedule of meals, you might be putting your body on grave danger. Intermittent fasting is not only about the concept of food abstinence. There are specific guidelines to follow to get more benefits. Luckily, experts have created several methods for successful intermittent fasting. These schedules will help you assess what schedule of fasting and eating is suitable for your body. In this segment, I will be discussing 15 types of intermittent fasting to choose from. It is advised to start from the basic methods to gain experience as you go along with the process.

1. 24-Hour Fasting

From the name itself, this method of intermittent fasting allows you to fast for 24 hours before having a meal. However, for people who are not yet as experienced in fasting, this is not advisable. The only time you should engage in 24-hour fasting is when you have finally established your body and mind to longer fasts. Without ample experience in fasting, you might be doing more harm than good to your body, especially when it is not used to abstaining from food at this particular amount of time. In this process, you can even eat at the 23rd hour and take in food for one hour to impose a higher calorie deficit.

2. 16/8 Intermittent Fasting

This type of fasting has been popularized by Martin Borkhan of Leangains. It optimizes weight loss with heavy and strenuous exercise. The concept is simple: you abstain from food for 16 hours and then eat within 8 hours. The number of meals you have for the day or week is not relevant in this kind of intermittent fasting. For this method, most people choose to skip breakfast and eat around noon. Therefore, they have an exact 16 hours from dinner until noon before they can eat at a time frame of exactly 8 hours. Others stop eating at around 8 P.M. and resume eating from 12 P.M. the next day until 7 P.M. For them, it is the perfect time to fast - and the easiest one at that. I, on the other hand, stop eating at around 6 P.M. onwards and resume eating at 10 A.M. the next day. When I have so much work to do, I get hungry in the morning. So, instead of waiting at 12 P.M., I eat at 10 A.M.

3. The Warrior Diet

This originated from the ancient four years like the Spartans in Rome who would stay physically active the entire day and only eat at night. During daylight, they were not allowed to eat because they were too preoccupied in building barracks and fortresses, including equipment for their beloved country. The only thing that helped them acquire the energy they needed for strength and stamina was beer, which was totally permitted for intermittent fasting. Evening was the only time they were allowed to eat huge portions of foods such as stew, meat, bread, and other varieties.

4. OMAD

OMAD is more popularly known as One Meal a Day. I am sure that most of you might have heard the saying, "An apple a day keeps the doctor away." But according to our father of medicine, Hippocrates, fasting is the best way to heal the body from illnesses. Hence, in this method, you will be fasting for about 21 to 23 hours and can merely eat for 1 to 3 hours. It doesn't matter which meal you eat as long as you are comfortable with the timeframe. If you have work to do in the morning, it is preferable to eat during breakfast and skip your meals until the next day. There are others who skip their breakfast and dinner and only eat lunch or brunch, whichever they see fit. Researchers believe that the method of eating once a day is ideal for losing fat but not for muscle growth. Apparently, fasting for 21 hours and above is enough to convert muscles into energy, which can be detrimental to other people.

5. 36-Hour Fasting

In earlier times, people can go for days without eating food. Nowadays, most doctors will not prescribe it. A person cannot even skip breakfast sometimes, let alone a snack during breaktime. Experts, however, have proven that fasting for over 24 hours can do wonders to the body. They have gathered that the longer you stay fasted and experience energy deprivation, the body is forced to trigger its longevity pathway to help mobilize fast, boost stem cells, and recycle worn-out cells. According to some studies, it takes at least one day to see significant effects of autophagy. But this process can be sped up by eating a low-carb diet before starting to fast and exercising on an empty stomach. Researchers also recommend using herbal teas to stimulate the process of autophagy. Unfortunately, such methods are not yet applicable for intermittent fasting enthusiasts. As mentioned a while back, it takes courage, determination, commitment, and self-discipline to accomplish this specific practice.

Before we move on to the next type of intermittent fasting, let us first discuss what autophagy is and what it means to the body. This is an internal process that aids in the destruction of dysfunctional cells. The term autophagy literally means "to eat itself." However, there is nothing to be alarmed about because it maintains homeostasis in the body by allowing the detoxification of bad substances to make way for cell regeneration. The purpose of autophagy is to balance the manufacture of cellular components and destroy the damaged cells and dysfunctional organelles. It may have seemed like a dangerous concept at first, it is needed by the body for healthier organs and skin.

6. 48-Hour Fasting

The 48-hour fasting is one of the most difficult forms of intermittent fasting. Once you've made it past the 36th hour, you can try this as well. A highly challenging part of this type of fasting is the adaptation phase in which the body is forced to cope with the changes it comes with. However, once you get used to the method, it will be easier to engage in more forms of fasting than the easiest ones. According to people who have experienced 48-hour fasting, they have reached ketosis faster, a state that activates autophagy. You will develop the ability to suppress hunger, feel mentally clear, and have a bit more energy and focus when you do so.

Like we said in the previous chapters, intermittent fasting can be a form of extended fasting when you chooses to increase the time of food abstinence. Still, based on a research, fasting up to the 24-hour mark is the most difficult battle to accomplish. If you want to commit this kind of strategy in the long run, you should train your mind and body to adjust to the physiological effects of extended fasting.

7. Extended Fasting

If you are wondering if there's something more exhausting than the 48-hour fasting, there is a method called extended fasting that can last for 3 to 7 days. According to several experiments, 72 hours of fasting can reset the immune system in their mice test subjects. The process generates blood cells in the body and promotes immunity. Fasting from 3 to 5 days is the optimal time frame for autophagy and prevents the onset of relapse among people. Although this type of fasting is not needed and ill-advised for some, it can do wonders for your body in terms of longevity, health, and immunity once you have accomplished this.

8. Alternate-Day Fasting

Alternate-day fasting is also known as the 5:2 diet as it allows consumption of approximately 500 calories on days when you can merely eat small portions of food during the eating window. By restricting your caloric intake, however, it makes the physiological effects of fasting more difficult to kick in. Plus, there's a greater tendency for you to miscalculate the number of calories taken during the day. Furthermore, there's a greater risk of losing self-discipline or trying to binge-eat.

9. Fasting Mimicking Diet

The ninth type of intermittent fasting is the fasting mimicking diet in which a person can eat 800 to 1000 calories a day for 2-5 days in a month. After that, you can return to a normal eating schedule starting from day 6. This type of intermittent fasting is known to reduce blood pressure, lower insulin level, and suppress IGF-1, which are all related to a person's longevity. When you follow this method, you're only allowed to eat foods with low protein, moderate carbs, and fats, such as mushroom soup, olives, nut bars, kale, and others. The idea is to make your caloric intake as low as possible and to avoid autophagy. But then again, there are downsides of doing this technique just like with alternate-day fasting.

10. Protein-Sparing Modified Diet

Protein-sparing modified diet is one of the least common forms of intermittent fasting. The method requires you to eat food with high protein content but low carbohydrates and fats. This is essential for bodybuilders who only want to lose weight and burn fat without the risk of autophagy. It also helps maintain leans muscles and make sure that you do not take more protein than what your body can take.

11. Fat Fasting

This form of intermittent fasting is known to be "fat fasting." Considering you have heard about the ketogenic diet, you should know that the effects of fasting and the keto diet are the same. It is only the methods that differ. Both of these facilitate the metabolic state of ketosis or the process of burning down fats when the liver no longer has glucose to spare for the body. This enables a person to acquire energy for the whole day. If you think that eating loads of fat will get your body out of ketosis, you are wrong. It might increase the amount of fat in your body, but it does not necessarily mean that the metabolic state will end.

12. Bone Broth Fasting

This is a method for intermittent fasting that allows you to extend fasting for a longer period of time. Bone broth contains amino acids that inhibit autophagy in the body. For fat loss, you will not want to consume large amounts of calories because it strips down the essence of losing weight. One cup of bone broth will suffice to give you the energy that you need to complete your daily activities. Furthermore, the electrolytes and minerals from bone broth are essential for preventing brain fog, lethargy, and muscle cramps.

13. Dry-Fasting

Dry-fasting is a form of intermittent fasting that prevents the intake of any form of liquid. This might be one of the most difficult types of fasting since most people cannot live without rehydration from time to time. Others, however, can live without solid food for days at a time with the assistance of water, juice, coffee, tea, and other beverages. However, there are only a few who can survive days without rehydrating their body. There is a theory that states that dry-fasting is equal to three days of water fasting. The concept is that when the body is deprived of any liquid, the body will start to reproduce its own by converting triglycerides from the adipose tissues or fats into metabolic water. Triglycerides are the main constituent of body fat in humans and animals.

Did you know that dry-fasting is a method of healing in some religious beliefs? This method includes restricted fasting for a time frame of 12 to 16 hours for maximum effects.

14. Juice Fasting

For a long time, I have never thought that juice fasting is a thing, but it really works! This method refers to using vegetables and fruits that ensure the intake of a significant amount of carbohydrates and fructose, which is essential in providing energy to the body. The idea of green and power smoothies can be associated with this kind of intermittent fasting. Researchers have found that someone can lose a significant amount of weight using juice fasting while promoting the buildup of lean muscle mass.

15. Time-Restricted Feeding

The last form of intermittent fasting is known as time-restricted feeding. This technique has originated from the popularization of circadian rhythms and chronobiology, which aims to restrict a person's daily food intake. According to further experiments, this type reduces the onset of metabolic disorders among humans and animals. On a more specific note, the mice that had been fed for eight hours did not get obese or develop any chronic disease as compared to those that were fed with the same number of calories without time restrictions. Simply put, when you aim to eat 1000 calories per day, avoid eating it in one sitting when you can diversify its intake in the span of 8 hours per day. Not only will this help you build a good sense of self-discipline but it will also boost your metabolism.

Chapter 3: The 30-Day Challenge

In the previous chapters, we have discussed the importance of fasting to people. Whether it is about weight loss, longevity or even prevention of several illnesses such as cardiovascular diseases, respiratory diseases, diabetes, and many more. When I first heard the idea of fasting, I honestly felt a bit skeptic about it. There were thoughts running within my mind saying that I might acquire ulcer from this or that I might develop more illnesses because the practice could crash my immune system. When I did some research, though, I was surprised to find out that the effects of fasting were quite the opposite.

The reason why I want to include a 30-day challenge for fasting is that it has really worked for me, given the right method of intermittent fasting. During the month of December 2018, it was inevitable to join several parties in a row. There was drinking and so much eating, especially during Christmas and New Year. It was difficult for me to abstain because I grew up in a family where social gatherings are very important. I couldn't simply decline their offer to eat because it would be rude. However, I engaged in voracious eating and drinking not because I couldn't say no but because I liked it. And I thought, "You only live once." That year was a rough one for me because I was diagnosed with nephritis or the inflammation of the nephrons in the kidney. Before that, I was diagnosed with angina and gastroesophageal reflux disorder. My doctor recommended having small amounts of food every now and then, especially when I felt like my stomach was building up too much acid. Eating and drinking excessively were detrimental, too. I was not allowed to consume food with salt or vinegar since they irritate the kidneys. This frustrated me during that holiday season, but I decided to do it because I was hard-headed. The downside was that everything got worse after the New Year when I felt every effect of the unhealthy lifestyle I emancipated last December. I grew stout and noticed a significant decline in my immune system. My parents thought that I was getting healthier. In fact, however, my situation got worse. So, I decided to fast.

Food abstinence was the most difficult challenge for me

because I was hungry all the time. To gain a little bit of self-control, therefore, I would distract myself every now and then. After days of research, I found out that there were other methods of fasting. Nevertheless, in my case, intermittent fasting worked the best to reduce weight and regain my healthy body. It was difficult to assess which specific tactic to use in fasting. But then, I realized that I had been doing it subconsciously even without scheduling or setting up alarms. After all, I was getting sick. My loss of appetite made me believe the concept of Hippocrates about food abstinence when a person was ill. From this, I decided to continue this 16/8 method for a whole month. Of course, in the beginning, I couldn't believe that it was possible. I thought that sooner or later, I would be tempted to eat a lot of food again. But as I ventured and persevered daily, I realized that I slowly developed control over my urges. I felt a sense of satiation, too, so I did not feel too hungry anymore unless my body would signal that it's time to eat.

After a month, I noticed a workable improvement in my health. I lost a couple of pounds, and I no longer felt pain on my lower back, which indicated kidney problems. At first, I thought that my GERD would worsen because of fasting. It turned out that, with the help of various healthy beverages, I was able to overcome this illness as well. Angina and heartburn did not bother me either. Thus, I did not intend to stop even when my 30-day challenge was already over.

Now, it is time for you to enjoy the same benefits that I do now by starting your own 30-day challenge. First and foremost, you need to assess the kind of method that you will be employing. You may refer to the types of intermittent fasting in the previous chapter if you are unsure of what to choose and figure out what is best for you. Furthermore, you should consider several factors.

1. Your Daily Schedule

Assess the time frame when you are free to eat. Base your intermittent fasting schedule to your work, school, and other daily activities. This way, your body will be able to adjust quickly with the changes. And if it is time to break your fast, you can maintain a healthy eat-fast period.

2.   Your Daily Routine

What are the tasks that you need to complete every day? The answer defines the time when you should eat. For example, you do heavy work in the morning, so it is best to have your meals as early as 6 A.M. before fasting after that.   However, if you are working late at night, it is advisable to eat at around 6 to 7 P.M. so that you'll have energy to get through your activities.

3.   Your Body Rhythm

Assess yourself and determine the hours when you feel hungriest. From this, you can schedule your eating periods on time and fast during the remaining hours of the day. Say, if you're used to skipping breakfast, you can start fasting at around 10 A.M. or lunchtime. In that way, you can successfully perform a full fast for the rest of the day or until your next eating period.

So, what should you expect when you start your 30-day challenge? Well, I am sure that we all experience the side effects of fasting on different notes. More often than not, though, the first week is the most challenging because this is when your body starts to adapt to the changes brought by food abstinence. The side effects may include headaches, bowel movements, cravings, and thirst, among others. Much like any other method, you will experience some drawbacks in the beginning. However, this shouldn't be something to be alarmed about. When you start noticing such effects, it is best to stay hydrated during most of the fasting hours. Once you go to work or school, you can bring water or green smoothies with you. This will help you develop a faster metabolism and speed up the process of autophagy.

During the second week, you may experience headaches as your body tries to accommodate your new diet. There's a greater need to satiate your thirst as well; that's why you need to have a lot of water. You can incorporate low-carb drinks such as grapefruit juice, cranberry juice, and other forms of healthy beverages. During the third week, you may feel the preliminary effects of intermittent fasting. You will start to lose weight and notice that you no longer crave for food as much as you have before fasting. You can feel a significant increase in your metabolism and mental sharpness. In the fourth week, your body will have accommodated the process and crave for intermittent fasting more. You will soon enjoy the effects of fasting such as alertness, better skin and hair health, enhanced immune system and metabolism, and, of course, a remarkable weight loss.

Chapter 4: Quick Start Guide

Now that you know what to look after while fasting intermittently, it is time to learn a quick guideline regarding the method. We have discussed in the previous chapter the several factors that you need to understand in order to schedule your new routine. In this chapter, we will be digging deeper into the different techniques to make intermittent fasting more convenient for you.

We all have different kinds of routines every day. As a worker, student, mother, or a pioneer, we always have to deal with a plethora of activities. Sometimes, no matter how much we try so much to engage in intermittent fasting, our schedule does not permit us to do so. Hence, it is very important to assess our time and foster self-management.

You read it right! You need self-management to make a successful intermittent fasting schedule. First and foremost, let us dig more into the term 'self-management.' In all honesty, I do not like to use the word "time-management" that often. Because, somehow, I believe that people cannot really manage time. There are 24 hours in a day, seven days in a week, and 365 and ¼ days in a year, and I do not think that you are equipped with the power to change it or at least slow it down. In truth, none of us can do that. This is merely a misconception from our end. The reality is that it is not the time that we manage; instead, it is ourselves and how we present ourselves to the circumstances of the restricted time, which allows us to manage our activities and finish things on time.

In this chapter, I will be discussing the importance of self-management when you are trying to do intermittent fasting successfully, as well as how you can manage yourself to be effective in your weight-loss journey. Self-management is known to be a vital factor when it comes to self-improvement and self-mastery. It empowers discovery, innovation, resourcefulness, and success in everything that you do. This term refers to how an individual behaves in whatever activity that he or she has to do. Self-management is very much associated with commitment, planning, decisiveness, productivity, and organization, all of which are essential to intermittent fasting. A person needs to learn how to manage himself or herself while emancipating a hint of motivation to support his or her ideas in the midst of any challenge. Self-management is also a manner of nurturing your personal network. When you can practice self-management, you may feel more inclined to understand your actions a little deeper. You may also become more willing than ever to accept and own up to your mistakes. Not to mention, you will be able to help people in the middle of any adversity, share your success to others, and pull them up for their own self-improvement.

It is easy to say that you have commitment and ability to manage yourself. However, it is way easier said than done. Most people in this world who have achieved success in their goals and dreams are reported to have a huge amount of self-management in their system. To develop this value, you need to apply simple steps in your daily living.

1. Stay Positive

"Think positive" - that's what many individuals always say. If I earn a penny every time I hear this short saying, I may already be living in a mansion now. Despite that observe and look at the people who genuinely embody positivity in their lives. These two words are not challenging to pronounce, but it is difficult to apply when push comes to shove, and the circumstances become too tough to handle. Why do you think this quote came to life in the first place? It is to provide a motivation to folks no matter how hard their trials may be. It is important to stay positive even when you have problems, and so you need to feel more inclined to think critically, decide, and solve problems efficiently. Maintaining a positive mind can reduce your anxiety, frustration, and stress, which are huge factors that brings down a person. Positivity prevents you from breaking down and giving up. It puts your issues in a new light, giving you hope that it is merely temporary. While you are trying to pull off a successful intermittent fasting schedule, it is inevitable to experience several forms of mishaps and shortcomings. However, when you think positively about your routine, you will see how easily these circumstances can be solved.

2. Learn to Manage Stress

There are people out there who deal with emotional breakdown in the midst of extreme stress. That's why you should learn how to manage yourself even when you are facing worries and anxiety. When people think about stress, they often see it negatively. In fact, there is a positive outcome of being stressed: it pushes a person to move forward and get things done. That is, if people know how to manage their minds during stressful moments. But when stress is present, and they think about it with pure negativity, they have a greater tendency to break down and stop trying. Stress and fasting do not add up peacefully in our system. When we are stressed, it is our first instinct to compensate for these feelings with sugary foods, which is something that we cannot do during our fasting hours. This might leave us hangry (or angry because of hunger). This is the reason why we need to learn how to manage these emotions. Here are a few hacks to manage yourself during stressful times.

Avoid Caffeine

Caffeine is known to increase the amount of cortisol in the body, which is responsible for increasing your stress levels. If you are a coffee person, it is recommended to shift your beverage preference to tea and juice from time to time, especially when you do not feel okay.

Stay Physically Active

Exercising is a good way to reduce your stress levels because it helps boost the endorphins or "feel-good" hormone in the body.

Learn to Distract Yourself

When you are feeling stressed, do not make matters worse by engaging in strenuous work. You know yourself too well. You have an idea when you are getting stressed out. Thus, you should distract yourself with other activities that can alleviate the tension in your body. Learn to rest when you get a break time; go out and enjoy the fresh air every now and then.

Acknowledge Your Emotions

There are instances when we fail to acknowledge our emotions, primarily when we feel stressed or frustrated. Neglecting or repressing your feelings and thoughts, however, can worsen your situation. The main reason why people experience burnout is that the cramped-up emotions are buried within their hearts. It only takes one emotional trigger to unleash all of them at once, and it can take a toll on your psychological and social well-being. So, whenever you feel stressed, let it out immediately. Never invalidate your feelings just because it seems negative. Embrace it and allow it to be a part of you. This way, you will understand yourself more and be able to live better and let things go easier.

Talk to People

One of the most important ways to destress is to talk to people about random things. You can open up to them regarding your darkest secrets if you want. Nevertheless, by surrounding yourself with happy people, you get injected with the happy serum as well. You start to see things differently and feel happy about yourself.

Be Responsible for Your Actions

Another common mistake is blaming other people and events for their mistakes and shortcomings. When you aim to become efficient at managing yourself, you need to start to own up to your mistakes and learn from them instead of pointing your finger to every other person on the planet except for yourself. Think of it this way: would you rather remain stagnant by pointing fingers at each other or stay productive and search for a solution?

Avoid Procrastinating

Procrastination is like a black hole that dulls the mind and lessens the motivation of a person. It is one of the most dangerous pits that no one can normally rise from. Whenever you feel the need to stay lazy, get up and do something about it. Never let your dull emotions cloud your rationality, especially if you have a goal to achieve. This is also a common problem among people who are trying to lose weight. Instead of going to the gym or doing home workouts, they choose to be a couch potato. Procrastination tells the mind that a certain activity is "so difficult" even when it is manageable.

Watch out for this type of issue! It can destroy all of your routines, including intermittent fasting.

Do Not Wait for Monday

Start now! Do not wait for the right moment to start. If you want to do something, do it already. How sure are you that you will be as motivated on Monday? Do not entertain the "what-if" questions in your head because they will cause you to fail. Instead, use your current drive to make the first step.

How to Schedule Your Fasting

1. Stay Focused on Your Goals

It helps to have a daily reminder of your goals and objectives every now and then. Remember when I told you to keep a journal? It is best to have it with you all the time to have a physical remembrance of the schedule that you should follow for intermittent fasting. As much as possible, avoid any activity that can derail you from doing the routine. Realize its temporariness so that you can withstand any challenge that life may throw at you.

2. Use a Calendar

Utilize the calendar feature on your phone or computer. You can even acquire a hard copy of the calendar where you can write your upcoming events and organize your agendas beforehand. Having one for intermittent fasting can help you track your progress during a 30-day challenge as well. For example, mark the days green when you have successfully employed intermittent fasting. At the same time, indicate what you felt, what you ate, and what you plan to do the next day. You can also have a customized calendar where you can write motivational quotes and boost your energy. When you think you have failed for the day, mark your calendar orange or red and mention the challenges that you have faced. However, instead of feeling guilty, use these shortcomings as a mode of learning for future reference. Indicate the solutions that you can try, to be specific, when dire situations come up so that you will not repeat the same mistakes again.

3. Use an Alarm

It is best to set your alarm 10 to 15 minutes before

breaking your fast. This is to ready yourself for the food that you are about to eat. It helps you to set your mindset and gain control over the next activities. Another advantage of keeping an alarm is that when your body has finally accustomed to the specific time to eat and fast, it can become your own alarm clock. It will synchronize itself and allow you to stick to an effective schedule of eating and fasting. This way, you no longer have to set an alarm, and your body will always be alert.

4. Schedule Fast Breaks

Schedule your fast breaks accordingly. Whether you are a worker or a student, after all, there is a specific time when you can get some lunch or rest from your activities within the day. To make fasting a lot easier to adopt, you can set your breaks during this time to avoid any hindrances in your daily activities.

5. Plan Ahead of Time

Most people disregard the importance of planning ahead of time. In fact, this method will allow you to schedule your tasks more successfully. It is best to plan things one day before it happens. For example, for my fasting routine for tomorrow, I will eat avocado at 10 A.M. as a snack. I might be able to grab some on the way to work as well. When you set things one or two days before it happens, it allows your mind to settle with the idea of doing such an activity. So, when the time comes, you are less likely to procrastinate because your mind is already set to do it.

6.   Don't Waste Time

One of the main reasons why people have constricted time is their inability to ward off procrastination. The most dangerous word to think about when scheduling and trying to do self-management is 'later' since it comes with no sense of definiteness. It can take hours or days before a person can actually accomplish something if you always use this word. When you have the chance to do something at once, maximize your time to do so to be able to do more things in the future.

Chapter 5: Dos and Don'ts While Fasting Intermittently

Weight loss is something that you may think about if you feel too bad about the size of your body. Hence, you might start looking for different diets to try. According to the World Health Organization (WHO) in 2016, there were more than 1.9 billion people across the globe who were overweight. More than 650 million individuals, on the other hand, were obese, and this case had tripled in number since 1975. With a high number of people dealing with obesity, there are weight-loss programs that have been done in hopes of reducing this count. These plans have been developed to help someone achieve their ideal physique.

As we have discussed in the earlier chapters, some people use intermittent fasting for detoxification, treatment of several medical conditions, weight loss, and conformation to certain religious practices. For instance, the Muslims fast during Ramadan. Intermittent fasting is a diet regimen that involves alternating cycles of fasting and eating. In simpler terms, you make a mindful decision to skip meals on purpose when you follow this method. Generally, intermittent fasting means that an individual consumes calories during a specific time of the day and prefers not to eat an ample amount of food for a longer period. Aside from weight loss, studies also show that this can help improve your metabolic health and protect you against diseases. However, in order to maximize these benefits, you must be able to carry out intermittent fasting efficiently. There are some instances when people complain about the lack of effectiveness of the method. The reason is that that they are unable to execute the proper procedure of intermittent fasting. For this chapter, therefore, it seems important to discuss the dos and don'ts of intermittent fasting to help you get better results. There are other methods to be followed as well in order to execute such practice without sacrificing your health. As what many practitioners say, fasting is good as long as you know how to discipline yourself, when it should be done, and how to avoid abusing it.

The Dos of Intermittent Fasting

Make A Plan

Intermittent fasting comes with different options, such as 24-hour fasting, skipping meals for 16 hours or having one meal per day. It is best to know which mealtime planning is best for you and what method suits your body well. Other people talk with their doctor before deciding what technique what makes the most sense, and that's something that you should do as well.

Make Sure You Are Fit to Fast

Make sure that you are fit to fast to avoid sacrificing your health for this method. You should not even thinking of fasting if you are pregnant, lactating, diabetics, or below the age of 18. Of course, it is not recommendable to individuals with underlying medical problems or those who are taking prescription drugs to evade erratic reactions in the body.

Prepare Your Mind and Body

Guarantee that you are in good condition and have a well-rested mind and body before proceeding with the technique. It is important to be able to focus on your goal, your reason for fasting. Preparing your body and mind can allow you to sustain the time of fasting and not feel weak easily.

Drink Lots of Water

It is important to stay hydrated while fasting as well. Proper hydration can help restrain you from feeling hungry. Water fasting, to be specific, helps promote autophagy, a process wherein the body breaks down and recycles old parts of the cells that may potentially be dangerous. Keeping yourself hydrated can keep you going and prevent you from dealing with an empty stomach all the time.

Listen to Your Body

While intermittent fasting comes with many benefits, it is still important to listen to what your body is feeling. Getting dizzy or weak while fasting can affect your ability to be productive and complete your tasks. You should only fast you feel healthy so that the food restrictions will not stress you out or make you feel fatigued and irritated.

Be Patient

Sometimes, people start fasting and think about how badly they want to lose body fats. With this mindset, they tend to avoid eating for a day or at any time of the day and keep on skipping meals. When these folks can no longer stand their hunger, they try to restrict their caloric intake severely. Although you can be strict or mindful of your diet, you should also refrain from depriving yourself of food when you are allowed to eat. Keep in mind that there are always healthy options to choose from after your fasting time is over.

Eat Enough Protein

Registered dietitian Molly Devine said that most people should be able to consume adequate protein amounts during an eight-hour feeding window. When fasting, excellent sources of protein like beef, chicken and fish can be had for two meals to obtain enough protein for the body and prevent muscle wasting. It is important to aim for at least 4 to 6 ounces of protein daily. Some studies show that consuming around 30% of protein can significantly lessen your appetite. Therefore, eating some meat and other protein sources on fasting days can offset some of its side effects.

Eat Plenty of Whole Foods on Non-Fasting Days

Maintaining a healthy lifestyle on non-fasting days is recommended. It is necessary to eat plenty of whole foods like meat, fish, eggs, vegetables, and fruits when you are not fasting because healthy diets based on them are linked to a wide range of health benefits, including a reduced risk of cancer, heart disease, and other chronic illnesses. The author of *The Protein-Packed Breakfast Club,* Lauren Harris-Pincus, said that anyone attempting to lose weight should focus on nutrient-dense foods, such as fruits, veggies, whole grains, nuts, beans, seeds, dairy, and lean proteins. Eating these kinds of foods on non-fasting days will keep you on track.

Consider Taking Supplements

Taking supplements is advised if you fast regularly since there are essential nutrients that you may miss out when you depend on the foods that you consume. Eating fewer calories regularly can make it harder for you to meet your nutritional needs, you see. Therefore, it is necessary to supplement your diet with calcium, iron or any multivitamin to prevent mineral deficiencies.

Stay Physically Active

Doing exercise while intermittent fasting basically forces the body to shed fat, considering the latter process is controlled by the sympathetic nervous system (SNS), which gets activated by exercise and lack of food. A certain study found that fasting before aerobic training leads to both body weight and fat reduction. Eating before a workout, on the other hand, merely decreases your body weight. The combination of fasting and exercising maximizes the impact of cellular factors and catalysts (cyclic AMP and AMP Kinases), which force the breakdown of fat and glycogen for energy.

The Don'ts of Intermittent Fasting

While there are positive things to keep in mind while fasting intermittently, there are also ideas that you should avoid no matter what.

Fasting If You Have Health Conditions

It is important to consider a healthy condition when doing fasting. According to Anne Brock, who specializes in weight loss and diabetic education, those people with type 1 and 2 diabetes, children, teens, and pregnant or nursing women should avoid intermittent fasting. It is necessary to follow such a rule because doing so with an unhealthy body might lead to severe consequences. Instead of helping, this might worsen your health.

Don't Overindulge the Night Before

Avoid overindulging in a fatty meal such as fries or burgers before starting a fast. Instead, slow-burning nutrients are recommended to be supplemented to the body. Anne Brock has also said that it is advisable to get some carbohydrates, protein, and unsaturated fats in order to ensure that you are getting nutrient-dense foods rather than varieties that are rich in trans fats.

Don't Work Out Too Hard

Performing any high-intensity workouts during a fast should be avoided; instead, you should only do light to moderate exercises. One study states eating combining low-intensity workouts with 20% to 25% of the participants' regular calories for two days per week has resulted in superior weight loss compared to fasting or exercising alone. Nevertheless, it is important to make sure that you are getting 25% of the required calories daily so that your muscle mass will not deplete." It is quite difficult to expend energy that you do not regain through eating; that's why you have look for a suitable workout routine that matches your intermittent fasting to maximize the results.

Don't Stress Yourself Out

Your level of stress can increase while fasting because some hormones might be triggered when you think too much about getting fast results. Stress boosts your cortisol level, a certain hormone that stores fat and breaks down muscle. It will be beneficial to practice de-stressing techniques such as yoga, deep breathing or meditation. Make sure that it is not too strenuous if you decide to calm down by doing an exercise, too. After all, to be able to function throughout the day, you need to reserve your energy.

While intermittent fasting has been globally popularized as a method to lose weight and prepare a healthy meal plan, there are still factors to consider before doing it. Following the dos and don'ts above can make you feel more confident about fasting and making it more effective.

Chapter 6: Mothers' Guide to Intermittent Fasting

Gaining weight while you are pregnant is what most expectant mothers worry about. Although some moms tend to shrug off the idea of gaining wait, there are still women who feel too conscious about their physique and want to bring back their pre-pregnancy body immediately. Some go on exercise, while others merely do not have time to do so. Most mothers put the needs of their children first, so they might not be able to take care of themselves like they used to before having kids.

Researchers conducted a study on nearly 30,000 women who had given birth between one and four times and found out that most of them never got their pre-pregnancy body weight back after giving birth. Some studies reveal that moms find it difficult to lose weight after the delivery even with breastfeeding; thus, they continue to gain weight. Just two weeks after the birth of their children, 63% of all women wish to return to their pre-pregnancy size and shape. Not every mother knows about the risks of doing so, however. There are issues recorded about new moms who have developed low thyroid function during and after pregnancy, as well as sleeplessness and stress, and they have all contributed to postpartum weight gain.

An associate professor from the University of Michigan named Olga Yakusheva conducted a research about women gaining weight, too. She realized that the reason why many mothers have higher rates of weight gain is that there was a change in their lifestyle. Furthermore, the study showed that that typical age-related weight gain for women is about 1.94 pounds a year, while those females with toddlers garnered almost a full pound annually.

Despite the fact that a lot of mothers are contented with their current physique, some may still prefer to find ways to lose weight. In this case, diet may be the first choice. The problem is that the current weight-loss trend that has become popular over the years is intermittent fasting, a method that requires you to go in and out of fasting mode depending on the type that you decide to take on. Question is, is it advisable for you?

There are women who experience missed periods, metabolic disturbances, and even early onset of menopause when doing intermittent fasting. However, this fasting technique can work for some ladies, especially mothers. The important thing to really consider is how it should be done. There are certain ways to do it, so you have a few options in your hands. Because your children will always be your top priority, and you should attend to their needs, there are certain tips to be followed to help you schedule your fast more conveniently.

1. Choose the right fasting hours

As a mom, household chores can undoubtedly keep you busy. For working women, your workload can add to your priorities. Nevertheless, you can still aim to lose weight by choosing the right fasting hours. You should define your hunger patterns and up to what extent you can continue fasting. Remember that you do not have to deprive yourself of food and drinks if you think that you cannot handle it. Any time of the day that works best for you is recommended. Figuring out the right fasting hours for yourself will set you up for success.

2.   Determine the best fasting method

There are different fasting methods to choose from. Since mothers mostly do a lot of chores at home or office, you should merely focus on finding the right fasting technique. One popular practice is the 16/8 method wherein you need to fast for 16 hours each day and restrict your daily "eating window" to 8 hours. Another technique is the 5:2 diet wherein you have to consume 500 to 600 calories for 2 days per week and eat normally in the next 5 days. The eat-stop-eat method can also be done, although it entails that you have to do a 24-hour fast once or twice a week. Alternate-day fasting is a different technique that allows you to fast every other day, while the warrior diet lets you fast during the day and eat a huge meal at night. Spontaneous meal skipping, on the other hand, means that you can avoid eating whenever it feels convenient to you. It is not necessary to follow a structured intermittent fasting plan, but you have to consider the best method that you can handle. After, such a factor might affect your weight-loss goals, as well as your duties as a wife, mother or employee.

3.   Make healthy food choices

Fasting works best when healthy food choices are considered. Though you need to abstain from eating or drinking up to a certain period depending on the fasting method chosen, you should opt for healthy options when you can do either. The craving for fast food or comfort food can really take over and increase the difficulty of making such choices. Some healthy foods to consider while fasting are low-carb vegetables, nuts and seeds, smoothies, and fruits like berries and avocados. Mothers, in particular, must find the balance that is the best for them to lose the post-baby weight. If cutting carbs and adding more protein and fats to their diet can boost their energy level and fend off cravings, they should do that. By sticking to healthy food while fasting, it may allow you to see the results faster than ever.

4. Stay hydrated

Drinking lots of water is essential when you follow the intermittent fasting technique. As a mom, you should always stay hydrated to be able to function throughout the day. Water can promote a better flow of blood, cognition, and muscle and joint support during the regimen. Avoid consuming diet drinks, though, because they merely contain artificial sweeteners. Some studies have shown a potential links between artificial sweeteners, increased appetite, and over-consumption, and they wreak havoc on your insulin levels and set back the entire purpose of fasting.

5. Take multivitamins

Since most mothers have a lot of duties to deal with, be it at home or in the office, starving themselves might not be helpful because they risk having vitamin deficiency. A daily intake of multivitamins might be the key to staying healthy while fasting intermittently. A practical advice to some women, especially those who are still breastfeeding, is to continue taking the vitamins that your doctor recommends.

6. Get more sleep

It might be difficult for mothers with a newborn baby to get more sleep, but it is essential if you are eyeing to follow a weight-loss plan and get better results. If you cannot stay inactive for longer hours, at least try to get a better quality of rest. The reason is that sleep is interconnected with our hunger pattern. Doing intermittent fasting can make the brain more active, which leads to the difficulty of falling asleep. Thus, a sleep routine must be set. Your body might adjust to the new plan, so you will have time to self-contemplate and detoxify your body. The more rejuvenated you feel, the clearer your thinking pattern is and the deeper you should be able to sleep. To loosen up your muscles and help the detoxification process, you can get a massage before your bedtime. Alternatively, you may try drinking green tea or chamomile tea to calm your nerves at night.

7. Exercise

According to Chelsea Amengual, the manager of Fitness Programming & Nutrition at Virtual Health Partners at the time of writing this guide, it is possible that your body will start to break down muscle to use protein for fuel while exercising in a fasted state. Plus, you are more susceptible to hitting the wall at this moment, which means that you will have less energy to work out as hard or perform as well as you have done before. However, as you adjust to the new eating pattern, it is important to be reminded that your training must not be overdone. While exercising regularly, you should increase its intensity gradually so as not to shock the body. Some experts also recommend exercising immediately before breaking the fast to reap the greatest metabolic benefits. Mothers have certain exercise options to consider, too, such as walking, swimming, and yoga. You are free to try any or all of them to see what gives the most ideal results.

While some people only think about intermittent fasting as an essential weight-loss tool, it comes with other benefits, such as providing healthy metabolism, activating the "cleanup mode," improving cognitive skills and memory function, enhancing immunity, lowering inflammation, and boosting longevity genes. It is difficult to guarantee how well or badly the method will work for you. If you decide to give intermittent fasting a try, you must make sure to listen to your body's feedback because easing into this fasting technique by skipping a meal or two every day might lead to initial symptoms of hunger and discomfort. If the system refuses to respond positively and causes you to feel uncomfortably, it is better to accept it and move on to other programs. In the end, your well-being should be one of your top priorities. Mothers wanting to lose weight through fasting, in particular, should be more mindful of their body and not abuse it since the kids need them. This idea is especially true for moms with newborn babies. You ought to be physically, mentally, and emotionally healthy while fasting to garner better results and avoid sacrificing yourself.

Chapter 7: What to Eat While Doing Intermittent Fasting

Every woman on a diet is supposed to plan what meals to eat for a day ahead of time. However, the procedure cannot be the same if we start talking about intermittent fasting. For one, not everyone may be familiar of the technique, even though it merely involves abstaining from consuming foods and drinks for a certain period of time. Not only has it been practiced recently but our ancestors have tried fasting back then as well. While most people in the olden times prefer fasting for religious purposes, it is on this era that the has become a trend for health and fitness reasons. Losing weight is something that someone who feels heavier than usually will most likely aim to do with the help of some dietary actions, including fasting. So, you can tell that intermittent fasting is not merely a fad.

Now, despite choosing not to eat or drink while fasting, it does not necessarily mean that you no longer have a chance to consume anything throughout this period. Of course, you can still do it; otherwise, you will starve yourself and deprive your body of nutrients that come from healthy foods. Although we are on a dietary plan, we should know what varieties to eat and avoid. The main question here is: are you willing to drop the unhealthy foods and drinks you used to love in the name of fasting? Are you willing to give up burgers and fries and ice cream for quite some time? For people who do not like vegetables, this might be a rough patch for you. Giving up the things that make you happy can be quite a pain - that is true. However, with the right motivation, I believe you can survive the ordeal, especially if you want to shed extra pounds.

What should you eat while you are doing the intermittent fasting, you may ask? There are certain food varieties that have been found to be ideal for consumption when you follow this method. These foods and beverages are listed as follows:

Water

The most common advice for a person who is fasting intermittently is to drink lots of water to stay hydrated.

Promoting hydration helps our body to continue functioning throughout the day. As we go through a period of abstaining from food from 12 to 16 hours, you have no choice but to use up glycogen, the sugar stored in the liver, for energy. As this energy gets burned, the amount of electrolytes and fluids in the body will decrease significantly. We are always told to drink at least 8 glasses of water per day to prevent dehydration and promote a better flow of blood, cognition, and muscle and joint support while doing intermittent fasting. Water is always the best choice to drink all day long. If you are not a fan of water, a lemon can be added as flavor to your water, as well as cucumber or orange slices. However, do not use any artificially-sweetened water enhancers such as Crystal Light because this will wreak havoc on your insulin levels and may cause you to gain weight in the process.

Coffee

This beverage is known to be a calorie-free drink. It is suitable to get your blood flowing in the morning, and it is important to kick-start your day. While your stomach might get acidic when you drink coffee on an empty stomach, you can use the beverage as an alternative for soft drinks, which are filled with sugar. Did you know that black coffee can enhance the detoxification benefits of intermittent fasting? It can also improve your body's insulin sensitivity in the long run. Remember that you can drink coffee, provided that you do not mix cream, milk or sweeteners with it.

Minimally-Processed Foods

Carbohydrates can trigger someone on a diet, in the sense that whenever they hear this word, they most likely give an eerie reaction. Of course, too many carbs can genuinely have a negative impact on our body, especially when our goal is to lose weight. While fasting, it is essential to think strategically on how to get the adequate calories that you need without feeling overly full. Though it is advised to minimize the consumption of processed foods, there can be a time and place for such items like crackers, whole-grain bread, and bagels. These types of foods are more likely to be quickly digested; thus, they are recommendable as fast and easy fuel sources of our body. Other foods to consider can be bagged spinach, sliced vegetables, and roasted nuts, and they can be pre-prepped for convenience. These minimally processed foods can also help if you intend to exercise while fasting intermittently even when you are on the road.

Tea

Known as a health elixir in many ancient cultures, tea has been a powerhouse enhancer, especially for a intermittent fasting lifestyle. If your fast calls for no energy-source intake, which means avoid sugar, milk or cream on any of your beverages, tea is the next best thing to turn to. According to a 2018 study, unsweetened herbal teas have been used widely due to their hydrating effect. There are different types of tea to try during a fast, namely green, black, oolong and herbal. However, research has proven that green tea helps to suppress appetite and enhance weight loss. In general, tea can boost the effectiveness of intermittent fasting by promoting gut health, probiotic balance, and cellular detoxification.

Apple Cider Vinegar

Another great drink for fasting is apple cider vinegar, which has anti-bacterial and anti-inflammatory compounds that can combat various health issues. Although this product is acidic, it helps in balancing the body's pH levels. No calories are found in apple cider vinegar, but this has minerals like potassium, magnesium, and iron. This can also lower blood sugar level, improve digestion, eliminate bad bacteria, and stave off hunger.

Potatoes

Like bread, the body can digest white potatoes with minimal effort. When paired with a protein source, it becomes a perfect post-workout snack to refuel your hungry muscles and energy. Potatoes can be a good source of many vitamins and minerals, such as potassium and vitamin C, especially if you cook them with skin. This is also high in the water content when fresh, although a potato mainly composes of carbs and contains moderate amounts of protein and fiber (but almost no fat). Furthermore, another benefit of making potatoes a part of intermittent fasting is that once cooled, potatoes can form a resistant starch primer that can fuel the good bacteria in your gut.

Soybeans

Soybeans contain a number of health benefits that come from the nutrients, vitamins, and organic compounds, including a significant amount of dietary fiber and protein. Common to Asian diets, soybeans play an important role in cuisines as they have been consumed even thousands of years ago. According to the USDA National Nutrient Database, soybeans comprise of vitamin K, riboflavin, folate, vitamin B6, thiamin, and vitamin C. Moreover, they are also a good source of organic compounds and antioxidants, which further help in boosting your well-being. Soybeans mainly grow in Asia and South and North America. In addition to that, there is one active compound found in soybeans, a.k.a. the isoflavones, which has been demonstrated to inhibit UVB-induced cell damage and promote anti-aging.

Nuts and Seeds

While fasting, another source of energy can be nuts and seeds. They may include Macadamia nuts, flaxseed, Brazil nuts, chia seeds, walnuts, pecans, hemp seeds, hazelnuts, sesame seeds, pumpkin seeds, and almonds. Nuts and seeds are excellent sources for protein, and they are easy on the digestive tract. However, do not eat more than a handful of nuts and seeds at a time. The proper discipline of eating some sources of energy on fasting is still best to keep in mind.

Multivitamins

The reason why a lot of individuals prefer to do intermittent fasting to lose weight is that the approach requires less time to eat. However, one should know how to follow this method properly. For one, starving yourself by choice may not be have a good effect to your body. While we keep disregarding our source of energy by skipping meals, there might be a risk of vitamin deficiency while in a caloric deficit. Nevertheless, this does not mean that you have to take as many supplements as you can afford. It is merely advisable to take multivitamins at some point because your body might not function well if you fast too much. Though a multivitamin is not necessary with a balanced diet that consists of plenty of fruits and vegetables, life can get hectic, and a supplement can help fill the gaps.

Seafood

This food group is rich in B vitamins, potassium, and selenium. Although they are mostly carb-free, you need to understand that the carbohydrate content varies for different kinds of seafood. For intermittent fasting, here is carb count for every 100-gram serving of specific shellfishes:

- **Clams:** 5 grams

- **Mussels:** 7 grams

- **Octopus:** 4 grams

- **Oysters:** 4 grams

- **Squid:** 3 grams

Smoothies

A registered dietitian and natural foods chef based in New York named Miranda Hammer said that the key to making things healthy is striking the right balance of vegetables, fruits, protein, and fat. "The smoothie is a really great way to get all those foods in your body," she added. Creating homemade smoothies that are packed with fruits and vegetables, therefore, can be a great source of energy and give you different essential nutrients. Furthermore, smoothies have a lot of health benefits and seem trendy for people who are on a diet. They are also often given a vital part when it comes to cleansing and detoxifying. Thus, smoothies are essential when you are fasting.

Low-Carb Vegetables

A nutritionist at Middleberg Nutrition in New York City whose name is Pegah Jalali once mentioned that low-carb vegetables are rich in fiber, vitamins, minerals, antioxidants, and many more. They also make a great vehicle for fats. The vegetables are considered a cornerstone of a low-carb diet, but one should take note of the correct varieties to consume. Overall, choose vegetables that are less sweet and starchy. The opposite of those are carrots, yams, beets, and turnips.

The foods and drinks mentioned above are probably the most recommended options if you need to top up your energy while fasting. Along with these are cheese, eggs, coconut oil, Greek yogurt, olive oil, berries, dark chocolate, and cocoa powder. It requires a strict amount of discipline and focus on your goal to realize why you are doing it. With moderation and self-discipline, you can enjoy these foods without suffering from the consequences that come with an ineffective weight-loss plan. Intermittent fasting comes with multi-health benefits, but eating something is needed to allow our body to function well throughout the fasting time. Furthermore, there are other recipes that you can prepare during your fast breaks to ensure the balance of nutrients in your body without compromising the essence of intermittent fasting.

William Cole, a Functional Medicine professor, recommends various recipes that you can try while fasting intermittently. In his segment, he has included simple meal preparations for your daily venture on intermittent fasting. For breakfast, for instance you can make a green smoothie. This can help to hype up your energy with a low-calorie drink rather than using a powdered fruit smoothie. You can use these following ingredients:

- 1 avocado

- 1 cup coconut milk

- 1 small handful of blueberries

- 1 cup spinach, kale, and orchard

If you plan to eat at lunch, you can prepare a healthy veggie burger to control your caloric intake and provide the energy that you need for the rest of the day. The recipe calls for:

- ½ pound ground grass-fed beef liver

- ½ pound ground grass-fed beef

97

- ½ teaspoon garlic powder

- ½ teaspoon cumin powder

- Sea salt and pepper to taste

- Cooking oil of your choice

Method:

1. Mix all ingredients together in a bowl and form the desired size of patties.

2. Heat cooking oil over skillet on medium-high heat.

3. Cook burgers in a skillet until desired doneness.

4. Store the burgers in a container in the fridge and use within 4 days.

If you are looking for a way to spice up your snacks, you can prepare cinnamon roll fat bombs. They are best eaten around 2:30 or 3 o'clock in the afternoon. The ingredients are:

- ½ cup coconut cream

- 1 teaspoon cinnamon

- 1 tablespoon coconut oil

- 2 tablespoons almond butter

Method:

1. Mix coconut cream and ½ teaspoon of cinnamon together.

2. Line an 8-by-8-inch square pan with parchment paper, and then spread the coconut cream and cinnamon mixture at the bottom.

3. Mix the remaining half a teaspoon of cinnamon with coconut oil and almond butter. Spread it over the first layer in the pan.

4. Freeze the snack for 10 minutes before cutting it into squares or bars.

There are also people who prefer to eat at dinner from 5:30 P.M. to 7:00 P.M. If you are one of them, you can prepare a salmon with veggies easily. Here are the ingredients that you need:

- 1-pound salmon or other fish of choice

- 2 tablespoons fresh lemon juice

- 2 tablespoons ghee

- 4 cloves garlic, finely diced

Method:

1. Preheat the oven to 400°F, and then mix together lemon juice, ghee, and garlic.

2. Place salmon in foil and pour the mixture over the top.

3. Wrap the salmon with the foil and place it on a baking sheet.

4. Bake for 15 minutes or until the salmon is cooked through.

5. If your oven size allows it, you can also roast your vegetables at the same time.

Chapter 8: Exercising and Intermittent Fasting

Exercise is a vital factor in your weight-loss journey. A regular workout routine matched with the power of intermittent fasting can help you maximize the benefits of both methods. When you stay physically active while fasting, after all, your body is forced to shed the fat that is detrimental to your health. It helps speed up the process of detoxification and autophagy as well, thus leaving your body rejuvenated, detoxified, and empowered. Despite that, too much exercise can affect you negatively. Like what we have discussed in the previous chapters, it is difficult to expend sugar and energy that your body does not have in the first place. According to researchers, when fasting and exercise are combined, it helps promote oxidative stress and prevent an increase of free radicals. According to Ori Hofmekler, a fitness expert, oxidative stress matters when it comes to maintaining your muscle mass. The condition not only makes you resilient to this acute kind of stress but also promotes the production of superoxide dismutase (SOD) and glutathione. Aside from that, it increase muscular capacity to utilize energy, generate force and resist fatigue. Thus, it is essential to schedule a daily workout routine to match your intermittent fasting plan.

When you exercise, though, you must eat food within 30 minutes after your workout. If you let the time go further than that, your body might break down and experience burnout, making you less inclined to finish your other activities.

Intermittent fasting is the process of limiting caloric intake through scheduling your meals at a certain timeframe. You can maximize the combined effects of fasting and exercise by scheduling your workout routine in the morning before you break your fast. This can help you increase your metabolism to a high degree. Not to mention, it is essential to kickstart your hormones and get you ready for a new day. Nonetheless, it feels equally important to listen to your instincts and be able to tell whether you need food before or after exercise.

In this chapter, I will be discussing the significance of

maintaining a daily workout routine in lieu of fasting, as well as the types that you can employ as you move forward to a successful weight-loss journey. In the meantime, however, let me discuss the different forms of workout that you can use to complement intermittent fasting.

Types of Exercises

Aerobics

Examples of this workout include swimming, dancing, and running, all of which are essential to strengthen your cardiovascular and respiratory systems. Apart from these, you can shed a tremendous amount of fat just by doing them from 15 to 30 minutes.

Strength

This is one of the most common forms of exercise. However, it is more popular among men than women, considering the program consists of weightlifting, doing push-ups and crunches, and using bodyweight to build muscle mass. Too much strength exercise during fasting is not recommended for some people. Without enough energy reserve, after all, the workout may damage the body. As mentioned above, if you plan to do strength training during intermittent fasting, it is best to eat within 30 minutes after your routine. Listen to your body when it tells you to stop; never force yourself to continue when you are already weary or tired.

Balance

This refers to the routines that help the body to acquire control and stability. A perfect example of it is yoga. This is the simplest, least extraneous, and most peaceful way to exercise and gain muscles. Even pregnant women are advised to practice it to increase their probability of having a normal birth. It allows for better relaxation and a stronger immune system. Imagine how much you can maximize its benefits when you combine this routine with intermittent fasting.

Flexibility

This is the form of exercise that allows you to stretch your muscles to improve your range and joint motion. Examples of these exercises include tai chi, water dance, yoga, and many others.

Why Should You Exercise?

Most people believe that when they are already fasting intermittently, they should no longer be required to exercise. Quite frankly, workout and fasting go hand in hand so that your well-being can improve. Remember that exercise is not merely about weight loss; it provides several advantages as well.

1. Strengthens Bones

Did you know that working out can increase your bone density and prevent osteoporosis? The latter is a condition in which the bones lose their density and are left to become weak and porous. It is most common among the elderly; that's why they are required to take a sufficient amount of calcium and maintain a regular exercise routine.

2. Prevents Cancer

Research has proven that exercise and fasting can reduce the onset of cancer among individuals.

3. Regulates Blood Pressure

As we have discussed earlier, fitness can promote the secretion of endorphins, which are essential when it comes to decreasing the level of cortisol in the body. If you have not noticed it yet, when people deal with an excessive amount of stress, they are more prone to having high blood pressure and hypertension, which can be dangerous for anyone.

4. Enhances Emotional Well-Being

Most people might not also be aware of it, but exercise can enhance your emotional health. Observe some individuals who are frustrated and depressed, for instance. They go to the gym instead of sulking in their houses and thinking about their day. A workout session can serve as a distraction to people who have a lot of thoughts that can cause distress. This process can help you obtain self-awareness and self-control. These are factors that are essential for maintaining a healthy psychological and emotional well-being.

5. Boosts Physical Health

Exercise, when combined with intermittent fasting, may allow you to maximize the benefits of holistic health. Together, they can strengthen the immune, cardiovascular, and respiratory systems. They can also inhibit the onset of stroke, atherosclerosis, apnea, and other diseases that you might acquire later in life.

Exercising While Fasting

After everything has been said and done, it is time to create your own workout routine to help you achieve your weight-loss goals. Remember that there is no specific time required for exercising as long as you have a regular way of doing it. If you feel like you are freer in the morning, you can workout for 15 to 30 minutes. However, if you are on a tight schedule during the day, you can do your routine before you go to sleep. Consider your daily activities while planning to avoid any time constraint that might stress you out more. Do not forget your situation and resources either. For instance, do you have a family to take care of? Are there possible distractions at home? Are you likely to exercise at the gym or home? If you're worried about the equipment needed for working out, you have nothing to fret about. There are exercises that do not require any tool except for your body weight. However, if you want to ante up your game, you might consider getting a gym membership and hiring a personal trainer. Be sure to inform whoever that individual may be that your fasting so that he or she knows what routines to suggest and ask you to avoid. If you choose to work out at home, you can utilize your gadgets to look for applications that can assist you digitally. You may also search for tutorial videos to watch; regardless if you are into Zumba or bodyweight training, you can always use the online experts' examples as a basis for exercising while fasting.

When you are a beginner when it comes to working out, you need to take things lightly during your first days of training, and then work your way up. Your body is very resilient. Even if you start at the low levels, it has the inclination to increase the intensity of the exercise as time passes by. Unknowingly, you will do more repetitions and sets than you have expected. From this, you will know that your exercise routine is totally worth it because it has significantly improved your stamina and agility in working out. Here are some tips to follow when exercising to lose weight.

1. Take note of routines that feel good to repeat.

I cannot tell you exactly what to add to your training program because we all have different preferences and body types. It is up to you to discover the forms of exercise that are fit for your body. In choosing these workouts, though, you need to make sure that you can execute the moves without causing injury on yourself. You must also consider the energy that you have left after fasting. Do not strain your muscles too much either. Let your body start from the easiest routines and adjust to it before moving on to the next level.

2. Remember to hydrate yourself every now and then.

If you want to break a sweat, you are going to need lots of water to facilitate the process of detoxification. This way, you can hasten your metabolic rate, as well as the burning of fats.

3. Learn to rest in between reps and sets.

Repetition is the number of times that you do a routine. For instance, 10 push-ups, 10 crunches or ten squats. A set, on the other hand, is the group of actions that you perform throughout the entire session. For example, one set may include 5 push-ups, 5 crunches, and five squats. You may say, "I did two sets of 15 repetitions of squats." That means that you have squatted 30 times. When you are in the middle of a workout routine, learn to rest your muscles every now and then or from 10 to 15 seconds after every action before moving forward to the next routine.

4. Do not exhaust the same muscles on the same day.

If you plan to start exercising now, you should decide on which muscle group to train first. Tomorrow, you need to choose a different muscle group, too. When you exhaust the same areas over and over, it may cause damage to the sheaths of muscles. Instead of having a lean muscle mass, its formation might become distorted and awkward to look at.

5. Perform warm-up exercises all the time.

This is one of the most important tips of working out: always learn to warm up for at least 5 minutes before an exercise to avoid any injury. This may include stretching, walking, or even cycling.

6. Utilize your distractions perfectly.

If you're so distracted with a television for the radio, for instance, you can use this to pump up your energy every time you are working out. It can also be a makeshift timer for your routines. If you get bored while doing so, you can turn on the TV and watch a show while performing the exercises. Meanwhile, when using the radio, you can use the songs or programs as cues for your routines. It may seem simple, but it is a very helpful tip to keep any distractions from getting in the way of your weight-loss goals.

Chapter 9: Effects of Having Malnutrition

People who pride themselves in being too fat often say, "This is who I am. Why should I change it?" Others quip, "I am contented and proud no matter what the weighing scale says." Although there is nothing wrong with accepting who you are, there is a deeper reason why you need to lose weight, especially if you have gone beyond your normal body mass index (BMI).

BMI is the measure of your body fat. If the value is normal, it means that the ratio of your height and weight is ideal. This usually entails that you are a healthy person with a healthy lifestyle. However, if your BMI is outside the healthy weight-height ratio, you are either malnourished or overweight, which can both lead to various diseases. When you fast, therefore, remember to check your body mass index regularly to avoid going below or above the normal value.

Before we start talking about malnutrition, though, let me discuss the essential fats that we need to clear out to prevent confusion and misrepresentation in the future. The first and most important term to recognize is adipose tissue, a.k.a. fat. This is the anatomical term for the loose connective tissues in the body that consist of adipocytes. Its role is to store energy in the form of fats that cushion and insulate the body. It also has four types, namely visceral fat, subcutaneous fat, fibrous fat, and cellulite.

Visceral fat is the kind of adipose tissue that is stored tightly between the organs in the abdominal cavity, including the liver, pancreas, and intestines. Too much visceral fat inside the body is the cause of a hard stomach (or "beer belly" to alcoholics). The more it accumulates, the more it pushes the abdomen outwards, which gives someone a remarkable gut. Luckily, for women, they are not as prone to storing visceral fat as men.

However, for us ladies, we are more prone to having **soft fat,** a.k.a. **subcutaneous fat**, which can be found close to the skin's surface. This kind of adipose tissue is very soft and rounded. Hence, its other term is "fluffy fat." The female hormones signal the body to hold onto these fats to prepare for several significant events such as pregnancy, menstruation, and puberty. This is the reason why we experience bloating and weight gain before any of them take place.

We also have **fibrous fat,** which is tougher and more difficult to get rid of than subcutaneous fat. One example of fibrous fat is the excess fat that shows around your bra. Due to the pressure from clothes, and other garments, fluffy fat becomes fibrous fats, making it challenging to burn and expend as energy for various forms of physical activity.

Cellulite is a term that most of us might have heard of. Did you know that 80% to 90% of women have cellulite in their system? These chains of adipose tissue accumulate in the bottom layers of the skin, and it worsens as people age. Cellulite is also known as the "orange-peel skin" because of its observable texture. It is usually found in the buttocks and thighs, but it can also occur in other areas. There are many factors that contribute to cellulite in the body. E.g., smoking, alcohol, lack of physical activity, tight garments and underwear, hormonal imbalance and genetics. Nevertheless, it doesn't mean that it cannot be fixed or prevented. We will get to that later.

Malnutrition and Obesity

Malnutrition can entail different things, although most people only refer to it as the lack of nutrients in the body. In truth, the term has two classifications, namely undernutrition and overnutrition. The former means that your body is not getting enough healthy foods; that's why it leads to serious illnesses like stunted growth, eye problems, diabetes, and heart disease. When a person is undernourished, he or she is likely to have a weak immune system that's supposed to ward off even the weakest bacteria or virus there is. Other symptoms of this kind of malnutrition are: hollow cheeks, sunken eyes, swollen stomach, dry hair and skin, delayed healing of wounds, and constant fatigue. In addition to that, did you know that undernutrition can cause depression and anxiety? When the body does not get enough nutrients that aid the production of serotonin, the individual tends to develop these psychological disorders. Serotonin, which is also known as the happy hormone, is one of the most important neurotransmitters out there, along with dopamine (the pleasure hormone) and endorphins (the feel-good hormone). Anorexia nervosa and schizophrenia are also linked to undernutrition because of loss of appetite, purging, and starvation.

Undernourished individuals lack common nutrients and minerals such as Vitamin A, which is essential in maintaining perfect eyesight. Undernourishment can also lead to enlarged thyroid glands and decreased the production of thyroid hormones due to the lack of iodine. They are deprived of zinc as well, a mineral that is responsible for appetite, growth, and healing. Iron is essential for brain functioning, regulating body temperature, and avoiding stomach problems such as the Kwashiorkor disease. This condition is characterized by a severe protein deficiency as well, causing fluid retention and a protruding abdomen. This is common among children in Africa.

The most common causes of undernutrition include

food insecurity, digestive problems (e.g., Crohn's disease), bacterial overgrowth in the intestines, and celiac disease. Excessive alcohol consumption is another reason for undernutrition in adults because the content of alcoholic beverages inhibit the intake of protein, calories, and micronutrients needed in the body.

Effects of Malnutrition

In every social media platform, we can see reports about undernourished people. Sometimes, when we go outside our homes, it is inevitable to see at least one homeless person looking for food. There are families who cannot eat within a day because they lack the resources to purchase what they need for their families. We see them and often ignore them. We do not even know what it really feels to have malnutrition. So, to further understand the importance of a healthy body, let us take a look at some of the effects of malnutrition in a person.

1.   Reduced muscle mass and low stamina

Malnutrition causes a person to be weak and fragile. You may find it difficult to perform regular activities and exercises because of it. When dealing with undernourishment, you may not have the energy and strength either to climb stairs, carry objects, walk far, and even stay awake.

2. Wounds take longer to heal

Lack of protein, vitamin C, zinc, carbohydrates, collagen, vitamin A, and other nutrients are needed for wound recovery. If you are malnourished, an injury takes more time to heal for you than for most people and might be subject to inflammation and infection.

3. Low immune system

Malnourished people easily get colds, cough, flu, and other illnesses because they lack the nutrients that boost their self-esteem.

4. Poor sex drive and fertility problems

When women try to conceive, it is important to develop a healthy body and change your lifestyle for the better. Without proper vitamins and minerals, this dream may be almost impossible for you to achieve.

5.   Difficulty in staying warm

This issue is due to lack of muscle tissues to ward off the cold. Fats keep us warm, especially during the cold weather. One of the reasons why many people die during winter is that they lack of supportive fats that envelop their bodies.

Factors Contributing to Weight Gain

Overnutrition, on the other hand, leads to overweight and obesity. People who are experiencing this condition are more likely to have inadequate intake of vitamins and minerals. For example, in a study of 285 adolescents, researchers have found that obese people have lower vitamins A and E at an approximate level of 2% to 10% than those with normal BMI. This is most likely because being overweight or obese is caused by too much consumption of processed, junk, and fatty foods with high calories but lacks the essential vitamins and minerals needed by the body. Apart from these, there are other factors that contribute to weight gain.

Developmental Determinants

From the term itself, the developmental determinants of weight gain refer to the "big moments" in a woman's life. One common example is the prenatal stage of a mother. Researchers have proven that mothers who have been declined of food and starved at the beginning of the first trimester are more prone to develop obesity, diabetes, and hypertension in their later years. Having a low birth weight is also associated with higher visceral adiposity in life, and it comes with a greater risk of cardiovascular and respiratory diseases.

The postnatal stage is also a factor in gaining weight. After recovery, there are some women let themselves go into binge-eating unhealthy foods, thus increasing the probability of being obese or overweight. You may have seen some mothers to significantly bloat after giving birth because they claim that they "have no reason" to maintain their sexy figure. To them, all that matters is they give what their child needs no matter what the cost is. They forget their daily exercise routine and the importance of having an inadequate amount of rest, which are both associated with increased weight.

Adiposity rebound is one of the most common causes of being overweight among children between the ages 5 to 7, too. This concept entails the significant increase of adipose tissues in children as they grow older. Researchers claim that this stage is the peak of growth in the youngsters. It is observed to be the years where they are most active, curious, innovative, and experimental in their surroundings. In turn, they will need a substantial source of energy; hence, they feel the need to eat more. Researchers have proven that kids who experience an adiposity rebound at earlier ages are more prone to developing obesity later. As we can observe in our own children, they are less active in their toddler years, and they have a little exercise to help burn the energy consumed for the day. Early adiposity rebound is attributed to advanced muscle and skeletal maturity of the kids, as well as the high protein intake of the parents during pregnancy.

Adolescence is another developmental stage that contributes to weight gain. This is the phase where adipose tissue deposition increases rapidly for some people. In which case, when a lady in her pre-adolescent period has too much body fat, chances are, it can increase remarkably during adolescence especially, with all the changes in her lifestyle and diet. Some even go through puberty and compensate its effects through eating and slacking off, thus causing more fats to stay within their system.

Adulthood is also a phase when you can gain extra pounds. As you perhaps know by experience, most of us have been physically active as teenagers. But as we grow up, we experience a sudden decline in physical activity. Plus, there is a gradual decrease of metabolism at this stage, slowing down absorption and breaking down of nutrients in the body. There are instances, on the other hand, when you may be too active in sports and other physical activities until early adulthood. When you stop doing all of that, there is a great probability for you to deal with bloating, especially when a high amount of food intake is not a complemented by physical exercise.

Genetic and Environmental Determinants

There are two factors that define the structure and personality of a person. Some studies that prove that the human genome is a significant factor for being overweight or obese. Researchers have found out that energy balance, metabolism, dietary components, and activity levels can be inherited from the parents. So, when a child is born in an overweight family, there is a huge chance that he or she might become one as well. Nevertheless, this should not stop you from trying your best to lose weight. Obesity might be in your genes, but it will not develop if you will not allow it to happen.

The second one is environmental factors. If you put yourself in a habitat where you can live a healthy lifestyle and prevent yourself from having obesity, then you are in a safe place. There is a concept in psychology called "learned helplessness," coined by Martin Seligman, to define people who have given up on their situation because they either are used to it or feel like they can never get out. This is characterized by low self-esteem, passivity, poor motivation, procrastination, and failure to ask for help. If you let yourself sink in this black hole, then you will not be able to make positive changes for your body.

A person's energy usage, which is also known as the energy expenditure, is divided into three main components, namely the resting metabolic rate (RMR), thermic effect of feeding, and energy expended for physical activity.

The resting metabolic rate is defined as the energy used or expended when a person is at rest, e.g., sleeping, sitting down, or doing other neutral tasks. When your RMR is too low, then there is a higher probability for you to be overweight and obese. The thermic effect of feeding, on the other hand, refers to the increase of energy expenditure after a meal is consumed. Lastly, the energy expended for physical activity, including involuntary movements, such as shivering, fidgeting, and posture control, is a vital factor to determine the weight lost and gained by an individual. When all of these factors are very low in rate, you are more likely to be overweight than not. You will need a strenuous amount of physical exercise and to pay more attention to their diet to solve this issue.

Smoking and alcohol also play a role in weight gain. Cigarette smoking gradually decreases the metabolic rate and limits food intake of a person. When you quit smoking out of the blue, the consequences fall back to gaining extra pounds. Meanwhile, did you know that excess alcohol in the body, when unused, gets stored as fat? This is the reason why drunkards develop what is commonly known as "beer belly."

There are also drugs that contribute to bloating and weight gain. Glucocorticoids, such as prednisone, hypoglycemic agents like insulin, and anti-allergens can have an impact on the matter. Other drugs, namely hormone therapy and contraceptives, anti-seizure drugs, antidepressants, and heartburn medication, may cause you to gain weight as well. Because these chemicals may contain stimulants that can hype your diet, your metabolism rate can decrease, thus preventing your body from burning sugars and calories at a higher pace.

Chapter 10: Intermittent Fasting While Menstruating

As much as we hate to have our period sometimes, it is a natural and necessary process that women deal with every month. We all know that menstruation occurs when an egg cell is not fertilized by a sperm cell. Despite that, some of us still do not know the main effects of menstruation on the body. In truth, it is a cleansing mechanism that flushes out toxins and other substances in the body. As you may have observed after a menstruation cycle, your skin becomes clearer and more refined than before. The reason is that the foreign bodies that we constantly take in are eliminated through the blood that we expel by menstruating.

However, we cannot help to think about the effects of fasting while you are on your period. Is it even okay to fast while menstruating, or do you need to stop for a while? What are the effects of fasting before and during menstruation? We need to know these things for sure.

According to experts, fasting is like menstruation, in the

sense that they are both natural processes. There are times when women do not have an appetite before, during or after menstruating, depending on your body's mechanism. Furthermore, the two methods can cleanse and regenerate the system to make new cells. However, there are instances when women experience pain and difficulty during menstruation. Some even deal with hemorrhagic anemia, a condition that takes place due to excessive menstruation. If this happens, the situation might worsen if you still decide to continue fasting.

Let us take a look at the few people who believe in fasting - the Muslims. It is no secret that during Ramadan, they mostly fast and pray. Nevertheless, what will occur if a woman is on her period? Will she be allowed to fast? According to Rose Khan, a 20-year-old Muslim, the menstruating women are excused from fasting during this time. Since menstruation is already a form of cleansing - and a way to lose nutrients, for that matter - fasting might overdo the process. The Muslim folks believes that although it is sacred to fast during the holy month for them, they must always consider the safety of their people first. Hence, allowing the females to skip fasting while on the period is reasonable. It shows that they understand that some women experience heavy and painful menstruations; that's why they cannot fast even if they want to.

There are several factors that govern a woman's menstrual cycle. It includes stress levels, energy levels, nutritional intake, and caloric intake, all of which are affected by intermittent fasting. We have discussed that one downside of intermittent fasting is the cessation of the normal functioning of some organs. Doctors have reported as well that the women who fast may experience irregularities in their periods. The truth is that this usually happens when a person fasts excessively without guidance. Thus, it matters to carry over the procedures effectively to avoid these shortcomings.

Nonetheless, if you are determined to fast on your period, there is a way for you to avoid burnout and fatigue during those days. To ease your worries, you should know that there are some people who benefit from fasting while menstruating. In a certain study, women with polycystic ovary syndrome (PCOS) have shown that fasting during a period gradually decreases stress levels and has limited effects on follicle-stimulating and luteinizing hormones. For overweight and obese females, fasting during menstruation has also been reported to cause a significant weight loss and decrease the onset of inflammation in the body. Before you fast on your period, though, have yourself checked up first. As long as your OB-GYN doctor says that you are fit to fast, I do not see why you cannot do it. However, to apply intermittent fasting while menstruating, you are going to need a less extreme way to fast and lessen your caloric intake. As much as possible, avoid the fasting schedules that can deprive your body of nutrients and minerals. Stay away from routines as well that allow you to acquire hypoglycemia or low blood sugar. Apart from these, here are some tips to remember when you decide to continue fasting during your menstruation.

How to Fast While Menstruating

Rehydrate Your Body

We have previously discussed the different beverages that you can drink to break your fast. It includes water, tea, and coffee. These liquids can help you boost the level of antioxidants in the body and cleanse away the foreign, harmful, and unnecessary substances that may be lurking in there.

Take Multivitamins

Taking iron-rich vitamins can help you foster a more efficient menstrual cycle. To avoid anemia and other conditions, you need to have sufficient levels of iron and vitamins C and B-complex. These minerals will help you ensure that your energy does not fall short while fasting on your period.

Listen to Your Body's Needs

Whenever your body signals you something, you should never ignore it. If it tells you that it needs a bit more sugar, it means that it needs as much energy it can get from foods. Give your body some time to revitalize and recharge during your period. Having more amount of sugar and calories in your body will not hurt your fasting protocol since the cycle will take care of these extra fats for you.

Avoid Strenuous and Stressful Activities

To avoid menstrual cramps and fatigue, it is best to lay off difficult activities for the week until your body is strong enough to carry over these activities. If you want to exercise, you may do so as long as you know your body can expend the energy that you need for your activities. If you cannot, you can compensate for the lack of exercise by walking short distances or meditating.

Keep Your Fasting Periods Short

When you are menstruating, you should avoid fasting for more than 12 hours. For a more efficient plan, you can choose the 5:2, 6:1 or 16:8 pattern, provided that your body has enough energy for your other activities.

Chapter 11: Intermittent Fasting for Women Over 40

Who said that women cannot fast when they go beyond the age of 40? I mean, a lean and healthy body is not limited to the young ones. They can also be acquired by our mothers, aunts, and even grandmothers. There are many people over 40 years old who have gained the body that they deserve to have. As we have discussed previously, there are various advantages of fasting that the ladies can follow, so you can achieve your fitness goals regardless of your age.

Detoxification is one of the effects of intermittent fasting that is needed by people over 40 years old, especially the women. Over the course of your lifetime, after all, your body has been subject to various environmental changes. You may have also been taking in several harmful substances that can affect the immune system and cause several illnesses as you grow old. When you fast, they can reduce the effects of these environmental factors and cleanse the body from the inside out.

Autophagy is also a process that works best for women about 40 years old. As mentioned in the past chapters, it involves the destruction of worn-out and dysfunctional cells. During intermittent fasting, you are more likely to experience a positive change in your skin and hair, making it more supple, radiant, and beautiful from deep within. The same is true with your internal organs. As we all know, they are composed of cells as well. Effective intermittent fasting will allow these organs to rejuvenate and become as good as new. This fosters a stronger cardiovascular system, respiratory system, reproductive system, and digestive system. Not to mention, intermittent fasting can help you avoid the stressful circumstances that you might encounter during the menopausal stage. This process is extremely vital, therefore, to help your body regenerate the integrity of its internal aspects and make you healthier than ever.

For example, for women who have acquired bad habits such as drinking alcohol and smoking cigarettes, intermittent fasting allows the cells in your kidneys, lungs, liver, and heart to get better, unless the substances have caused enough damage to the organs to the point of no return. How amazing is it to develop a perfect and healthy body even at 40 years old?

Nonetheless, there are fasting disadvantages that you should know about at this stage. You might already be aware that as you get older, your immune system becomes weaker as well. This makes the body prone to several diseases such as cardiovascular disease, diabetes, osteoporosis, and many more. If you cannot obtain a sufficient amount of nutrients to ward off these kinds of illnesses, then you will be putting your body in grave danger. Before you engage in intermittent fasting at 40 or above, therefore, you should consult your doctor about it first. And if you are very much determined to try intermittent fasting at this age, there are some tips to remember to maximize the effects of this process.

Fasting Tips for Women Over 40 Years Old

Ask Yourself Why

There are a lot of people who remain skeptic when they hear about the magic of intermittent fasting as it can help someone lose weight and obtain a healthy body. As a woman over 40, you need to rethink your priorities, as well as decisions to engage in intermittent fasting before you start. Are you really ready for this? Why do you need this? What can you gain from it? After answering these questions honestly, you can get motivated to develop a healthy lifestyle as the time passes by. It allows you to have self-control and be able to ward off any temptation to overeat and try harmful activities. Without that, you are bound to fail in your attempt to acquire a healthy body. So, stay true to yourself. If you start intermittent fasting without commitment, you will only be wasting your time.

Apply the Golden Rules of Weight Loss

The golden rules of weight loss at the age of 40 require you to eat less by cutting back your meal portions, aim to lose 1 to 2 pounds per week, and remember that skipping meals will mess with your metabolism. Ironic, isn't it? For younger people, it is totally normal to forgo breakfast or any other meal of the day to follow an intermittent fasting schedule successfully. However, for women who are aged 40 years old and above, skipping meals can totally cause a decline in your metabolism; that's why you should merely consume fewer calories in a more frequent manner. We will discuss it later in this segment.

Rethink Your Nutrient Intake

Another tip for fasting when you are 40 years old is to always keep your carbohydrate intake in check. It is advisable to add more protein to your diet to avoid muscle loss, as well as speed up your metabolism. In your diet, you must have fruits and vegetables, as well as lean protein from Greek yogurt, eggs, chicken, and fish. Also, when you do grocery shopping, make sure to include whole grains, beans, and other healthy foods on your list. Furthermore, did you know that fats are essential to improve muscle mass and bone density? To do this without stripping the essence of intermittent fasting, aim for 7 to 10 grams of fat every time that you have it on the table. That is approximately about 1 ½ teaspoons of olive oil, ¼ of avocado, and two tablespoons of nuts and seeds.

Do Not Forget to Stay Physically Active

As we have discussed in the earlier chapter, exercise and fasting are not bad at all together. To maximize the benefits of these two methods, you need to observe a regular routine every day. It doesn't matter what kind of exercise you do as long as it fits your body and will not possibly injure you. It can pertain to 15 or 30 minutes of walking every day or stretching in the morning; what matters is that you are moving and your muscles are working.

Eat Fewer Calories More Frequently

Researchers have found that as a person grows older,

their metabolic rate declines along with it. To slow down this process, it is recommended to eat fewer calories in a more frequent manner rather than eating foods with a high number of calories less frequently. The latter process is a common mistake when it comes to fasting. If you aim to speed up your metabolism and the process of autophagy, you are going to need a few calories in frequent doses.

Mind What You Eat

There is a famous saying that goes like, "You cannot teach old dogs new tricks." However, I beg to differ. The human mind is resilient no matter how old a person may become. I genuinely believe that the more you are, the more you are granted with self-control. To maximize the effects of intermittent fasting, you are going to need to learn to say no to certain foods even if you enjoy them so much. In case you want to lose weight or develop a healthy body, you need to be more careful of what you eat, as well as watch out for those choices that give you heart disease, diabetes, and other related conditions.

Avoid Alcohol and Cigarettes

Drinking alcohol and smoking cigarettes will nullify the true effects of intermittent fasting if you keep on doing them. As much as you love these activities, you have no choice but to quite on both for the sake of being healthier than ever. If you have been an alcoholic your whole life, it may be extremely difficult for you to abstain from these substance. However, little by little, if you gain a bit of self-control every day, you can ward off the temptation of drinking alcohol or smoking cigarettes. Think about your health 10 or 20 years from now. How sure are you that you have not developed lung cancer, liver cirrhosis, or other illnesses due to these vices around that time? This might be a hard pill to swallow, but you're not getting any younger. If you want to live longer, you're going to need to change your lifestyle not for your family or friends but for yourself. There is so much to live for and see in life. You wouldn't want to miss those golden years of yours when you reach 60 or 70. Other people love to go for a reason. They believe that the remaining years of your life are when you truly see the wonders that it can provide. Why should you miss that opportunity when you have the chance to reach it?

Plus, if you have a family, wouldn't you want to see your grandchildren grow and become successful individuals in the future? Wouldn't you want to experience them pampering you, taking you to places you have never thought you can go to, and eating food that you have never tasted in your life? These little things matter as you grow older. Nevertheless, as you do, I hope you don't get a lot stronger and wiser.

Chapter 12: Common Mistakes When Doing Intermittent Fasting

You must have known by now that intermittent fasting is a tricky method for losing weight. You need to discover what your body really needs in order to experience and maximize the benefits of the process. What's risky about intermittent fasting is that there are several ways to do it and that there is no better way to find out which one suits you until you try them all. I am sure that you must have chosen a specific kind of fasting, and I totally hope it works for you. Now that you have established your goals towards successful intermittent fasting, you are now ready to start your journey and make your first step. But before you do that, you must furnish this information within your mind to avoid any setbacks or shortcomings during your fasting periods. In this chapter, I will be discussing the common mistakes that people do while intermittent fasting, as well as its effects on the body.

Being Too Hasty in Making Decisions

During the process of intermittent fasting, it is inevitable for people to feel like giving up. At times, they can no longer help but eat. The question underlying this problem is, "Are you sure that you cannot go any longer or is your drive making you say and think of these words?" This is one of the main reasons why I am promoting self-mastery and self-discipline. In order to engage in intermittent fasting and experience its effects fully, you need to be more committed to your chosen line of weight-loss method. Yes, when you are fasting, you will feel irritable, angry, depressed, and frustrated about your actions. Sometimes, you will even feel stupid for trying because you know deep inside that you cannot do it. Your mind will be scouring for reasons to stop. However, it is up to you if you let it stop you from losing weight and experiencing its various health effects. I cannot prevent it if you want to give up already; you make your own decisions. And as they say, "You are the captain of your own ship." But before you throw in the towel too soon, I want you to rethink your choices and remember why you started intermittent fasting in the first place.

Not Eating Enough

There are people who do intermittent fasting as a form of starvation. To them, they lose more weight without eating at all. They just don't know how much damage they cause to their bodies when they do not eat enough or at all. The reason why people drink during fasting is to avoid stomach, circulatory, kidney, and liver problems. When the body lacks the things it needs to function, it may cause detrimental effects to your overall death. This is what you need to watch out for. The people who fast for 36 hours experience more than what you do, and they have a way to distract themselves during fasting hours. So, do not try eating like a bird unless you want to get yourself in trouble.

Too much or Too Little Exercise

There is a rule called the 80/20 rule, which states that 100% of your progress relies on 80% diet and 20% exercise or physical activity. The 20% is a significant amount to maximize the effects of intermittent fasting in the body. However, make sure that you do not overwork yourself, especially when you are not getting enough energy from your fasting periods.

Forgetting to Drink

When your body is in a fasting state, it starts to break down and destroy dysfunctional and worn-out cells. In order to make the process effective, you're going to need to flush these toxins out by drinking water or tea or any healthy beverage of your choice. It is actually advised to drink about 4 to 5 liters per day, considering most of it gets consumed during fasting hours. Furthermore, drinking such fluids is the only way to compensate for the nutrients and energy that are needed by the body to perform several activities while fasting. Some people who engaged in intermittent fasting have been reported t0 sweat more during their fasting hours as well; that's why you cannot be dehydrated at all.

Forcing the Body to Fast

We have discussed earlier that there are people who are not advised to fast. When you are one of them, kindly stop forcing yourself to lose weight through fasting. I am sure that there are other ways to fulfill your need to lose weight and obtain a healthy body other than this method. If you insist on fasting, you will only be putting yourself in danger.

Making Excuses to Eat Junk

People with no self-control will always find a reason to eat what they want even if it is not a part of their fasting schedule. When I told you to listen to your body, I wanted you to be honest about the things that you feel and not make up a reason to break your fasting schedule. When you start doing the latter, your mind will be accustomed to the thought that it is okay and that no harm will come to you. The truth is, after everything that you have been through, it shocks me to find out that you are willing to sacrifice your efforts just because of a temporary enticement. Remember that the most permanent thing in this world is change. You will not be fasting forever. Why can't you wait for the right moment to eat and do whatever you want? I just hope that when you start fasting, you will be serious about it. Or else, this book will be all for nothing.

Obsessing Over Intermittent Fasting

Finally, it is a mistake to let yourself get too obsessed with the process. When you allow yourself to be that way, you start to become dysfunctional in other activities. Your mind will revolve around the thought of intermittent fasting, which can be dangerous to your health. Being obsessed with the method tends to make you overfast, overcompensate, and overwork. This can cause burnout and extreme fatigue - two situations that can lead you to a hospital. Furthermore, when you get too obsessed with the process, there is a great tendency that you might experience depression every time that you fail to follow one of your schedules.

Let me clear up one thing. It is possible to develop a sense of self-mastery over your eating and fasting hours. However, it is okay to slip up from time to time. Committing mistakes and experiencing failures are normal parts of life. It makes us all human. So, live your life to the fullest while using intermittent fasting as a way to improve your lifestyle, live longer, and enjoy more of life's bounties.

Chapter 13: The Power of the Mind Matters

We have mentioned at the beginning that mindset is an important factor for successful intermittent fasting. This chapter is one of the most vitals segments since it discusses various ways to control your mind whenever you contemplate between eating and not eating. So, I would gladly talk about how you can train your mind to say NO to every temptation that you encounter in your daily life. If you are used to eating more than three times a day, for instance, it will undeniably difficult for you to comply at first to the fasting protocols. However, as you push yourself harder towards success, there is no turning back. Your mind will be trained to withstand any temptation no matter how delicious or aromatic the food in your surrounding may be. In order to gain full control over your mind and emotions, you need to understand your possible urges and the reasons why you feel the need to comply.

Obsession

Constantly thinking about foods that you should not have can reel you into giving in to temptations around you. It becomes unhealthy for the mind and the body to be obsessed with only one thing. Sooner or later, this will start to make you dysfunctional as a person. Rumination is the number one key to failure not only in intermittent fasting but in all aspects of life as well. When you find yourself thinking of eating over and over again, you ought to find a way to distract yourself through productive means.

Seeking Out the Action

Your body starts to crave for eating or drinking too much because your brain is hardwired into such an activity. In other words, it has become a hard habit to break. In these cases, you can try to compensate on similar but more healthy behavior. For example, your body is looking for food at around 10 in the morning, but it is not time to eat yet. Instead of taking in loads of food varieties, settle for beverages and workout. That way, you can find another reason to fast until the eating window starts. It makes your vision about losing weight more clearly and more achievable when you motivate your body to stay away from foods a little longer.

Compulsively Engaging in an Activity

The main problem with other people is their lack of self-control. When somebody asks them, they eventually agree and forget about their long-term goals. For this case, I want you to set your priorities straight. Think about the consequences that your actions are going to bring. What will you feel after you have eaten with your friends? Who have you fooled? It is not your friends whom you keep fooling but yourself. I do not mean to be blunt, but you will not finish anything successfully without the essence of self-discipline. So, before you say anything to anyone, give yourself time to think twice. These activities are just preliminary and temporary goals. They cannot help you in the long run. Focus on the length of your objectives and who you want to be in the future. I hope it helps you find the control you have buried within.

Withdrawal

When a person suddenly stops a recurring action, such as smoking, drinking, or eating from fast foods, it brings on issues like irritability, restlessness, and depression. Because of these feelings, you may become more inclined to give in to temptation; that's why you tend to seek out the same actions and get obsessed with getting back in the game.

Lack of Confidence

Self-confidence is one of the key factors to uphold in every goal, especially when you are fasting intermittently. Just by thinking "I cannot stop" or "I will not be able to accomplish it," you are already sentencing yourself to failure. So, before you engage in intermittent fasting or any other activity, make sure that you are emotionally prepared beforehand.

How to Have Self-Discipline While Fasting

Now, I will be teaching you how to have self-discipline in the midst of a difficult challenge. Imagine this: you are invited to a party, and you have no choice but to say yes. At the gathering, there are food and wine. It is impossible to restrain yourself from all the drooling over the varieties laid on the table. They have even managed to make all your favorite foods. Your mind and body are scouring for a way to convince your mind to go through with it. However, you know that you should never let your emotions guide your actions. So, what will you do then?

First, I want you to close your eyes and breathe. You can go to the comfort room for a moment if you want to. From there, you need to visualize your goals clearly. What do you want to do? Do you want to eat? Why do you want to eat? The common answers are, "I want to try the foods because they seem so delicious" and "Forget intermittent fasting; I will only live once, and today is my cheat day" (even when it is not). It can also be, "I cannot take it anymore. My friends are eating, and it will be rude to say no when somebody offers me food!"

In reality, these are just made-up reasons from your subconscious that tells you that you should eat. When you give in to the temptation, it means that your emotions have more control over your mind, which should never be the case. When you let your emotions take control of who you are, there are various repercussions that you are inclined to face, such as poor decision making, lack of problem-solving skills, and cowardice. You will not be able to live your life to the fullest by being emotionally driven. It is just a made-up reason because they no longer have control over the thoughts instilled by their pleasure principle. You need to learn how to separate your rational objectives from your basic drives. There are many ways to think rationally and bury these emotions.

While you are in a private spot, close your eyes and breathe deeply. Count from ten to one while thinking about other things, such as your breathing, what you are feeling, what you want to accomplish, and other stuff that may be standing in your way. Create a clear vision of your body and health goals as you breathe. Do not break your concentration. Just let the thought sink into your veins, giving you the power over your mind. Accept the emotions that you feel about not eating. Turn the frustrations into a ball in your mind and throw it away. Convince yourself that it is for the best. It is for your own good and benefit. Ask yourself, "Why should I waste a perfectly good streak right now?" Think about what you will feel if you eat. You will hate yourself for being too weak, too emotional. And you will regret having to binge-eat at the party.

Instead of looking inside yourself and searching for your emotions, ignore these drives and urges and turn it into control. Let your mind throw away the fear, pain, sorrow, and despair. Rather, see how much better you will be doing after you have finished your fasting routine. You want to wear your two-piece or one-piece bikini on the beach? Visualize that! Do you want to stop getting bullied because of your weight? Picture that out! Are you tired of all the names they have been calling you? Are you willing to accept that pain for the rest of your life? See, temporary pleasure does not account for a permanent and long-lasting change in your life. Do not be that person who lets herself commit a mistake and then wallows in regret after doing so. You know what they say: prevention is always better than cure. So, before you do something that you might regret, put yourself in a strong position where you can withstand the pressure of not eating.

How to Say No

The second issue is saying no to people who offer you food. The variety is already at your face, its aroma dancing around your nostrils like the devil in disguise. What do you do to say no so that no how much they offer to you, no matter how scrumptious they seem, you will not budge and give in? The main notion when you say no is the fear of offending the host and other guests for not eating. In truth, there is nothing to be afraid of or anxious about. After all, we are in the land of the free. As long as you pay your respect to everyone and converse with them graciously, you will not have a problem. They will not mind if you do not eat at all. If these people offer you food, they will not be offended when you say, "No, but thank you." If they ask you why, tell them that you are following a strict fasting schedule for health reasons. They will not demean you for that. In fact, they may even admire you for it. It takes courage to say no to a delicious meal. Just tell them you will only have tea or whatever drink they can offer. Granted, there will be individuals who will bash you for it, but who are they to think about? You are doing this for your own good, not theirs. When you are on the road to change, it is inevitable that some of your friends or family members will not be able to understand why you are doing this. Others might say that you have changed and that you have suddenly become a killjoy. But you need to make them realize that you are doing this to lose weight and improve yourself. You need to say no to the activities you have been excessively doing before, such as smoking, drinking alcohol, and even doing drugs. The hardest part is that intermittent fasting makes you say no to food. Do not expect everybody to understand what you need to change for yourself and why you want to change it. The people who are right for you will understand no matter what you decide to do. They will care about you and perhaps even help you in your weight-loss journey.

Furthermore, some individuals take it as a challenge to say no to other people because they are shy or nervous of getting rejected by the society. If they only knew the underlying reasons why you are fasting, then they will realize how important and difficult it is. Ignore the naysayers, as Arnold Schwarzenegger has said a million times. Focus on yourself and your health instead. Who cares about what they think? As long as your friends and family support and accept you for who you are, you do not need to get approval from anybody else. To say no to a person, you actually need to use the word and not beat around the bush. Avoid saying "I am not sure" or "I will think about it." When you really want to commit to decline, you have to say the magic word 'no.' So, here are some of the proven ways to say it without offending anyone.

The first one is to use firm but polite alternatives for the word. Use sentences such as "I appreciate it, but no, thank you" with a smile. You can also use the words, "Not today" or "I'm sorry, but I cannot. I'm not really into it. I think I will pass." When they ask you why, it is best to reply with a quick and subtle answer. If you go on and on about what you want to do, chances are, the asker will find a way to convince you and make you say yes. Make excuses such as, "I have a lot on my plate right now" or "I am too busy; I need to do a lot of things." Then, end your statement with another statement to change the topic or end your conversation by saying you have to go. You do not have to have an elaborate excuse for doing what you want. As long as you have made them understand that you want nothing to do with those activities, then you are good to go. When they ask you about it even more and try to reel you into agreeing, do not hesitate to say no as much as you can. Be as firm yet polite as you can be. No further reasons. However, there are instances when people can be very persuasive. So, before you get second thoughts into sticking with your intermittent fasting plan, think of the most rational explanation to tell them – something that they will believe and understand.

In other occasions, jokes work better than excuses. They won't even know that you are indeed joking. For example, when you are offered to eat at a party, you can just say, "No thanks, I am on a diet." Chances are, they will react in disbelief because of your statement. You already know what is in their minds. You can just manipulate them by saying, "I'm already overweight, I need to trim down fats" confidently. Why? Because it is the most rational reason for saying no. They will even push you to do better. If they ask you about it, then you can tell them about your methods - no more, no less. Maybe by doing so, you will be helping other people in staying fit and healthy as well.

There is a phrase that defines most people nowadays that is known as "disease to please." This concept defines people who do their best just to belong in a group. If it means saying yes to everything and breaking your values and vows, they will take it, especially when it grants them fame. People in this generation believe that fame is a new source of power. Strangely enough, to win the hearts of people easily, you need to be famous. Even in politics, winning is not defined by your political platform but your popularity among the people. This is the concept that you should totally avoid not only for the sake of your health but also for the sake of your psychological well-being. You do not have to please everyone. You do not have to say yes to everything. You only need to be yourself, and you will get through life with flying colors. Think of it this way: when you have the disease to please, you might jump off the cliff the moment your friends decide to do it. You will ruin your life just to be "in." Is that the lifestyle you have always dreamed of as a child? When you are on the road to a successful intermittent fasting plan, you are not only training your mind to say no to food. You are training yourself to say no to every unhealthy activity there is in the world. And by committing to this venture and making it a habit, you can change not only your lifestyle but your way of thinking as well.

You know your friends so well, so you can tell which one of them is a serial asker and good persuader. It is always best to ignore them and avoid getting in contact with them, especially when you know there are significant events coming up. You can say no even when they have not asked you yet. This concept is known as crystal balling. If you ever get into the topic with something you want to decline to, you can call ahead of time and avoid any more persuasions by saying no. You can then say, "I'm sorry but I do not have enough money to go" or "My mom and I have plans for the weekend, so I cannot go." If you want to be softer in your approach, you can say, "I wish I could go, but I already made plans with some of my other friends this weekend" or "I wish I could go, but I already spent my cash on something else." "It is an honor. But…" could also be a phrase to start it off, especially when you are dealing with respected people in the society. White lies cannot hurt anyone, especially when it is for your own good.

If you are feeling uncomfortable and unconfident about yourself, you tend to be less assertive. But this should not be the case. Overweight or not, you have a reason to believe and stay confident about your talents and yourself. You need to be confident about the magnificent powers you are showing to the world by deciding to fast just so you can have the body you have always wanted. If that is not enough to boost your self-esteem, think of the successes you have had in your life. I am sure that those experiences can account for your unique abilities and personality as an aspiring human being. On the road to holistic change, you are going to need assertiveness. Do not let other people push you around like you are a child. You have your own decisions to make. You have your own battles to fight, including your goal to have a healthy body and a healthy lifestyle. So, when you talk to people, try to assert yourself more. What do you want? What don't you want? It is time to change the era of always being the second choice, the one who is pushed around. You are a beautiful and amazing person. Do you know that? It is time to learn how to become more mindful in the midst of peer pressure, anxiety, and belongingness in the community.

Now that you know the many ways to say no to many people around you, it is time to apply what you have learned. Practice makes perfect. The hardest part of declining to do your beloved activities is the feeling of being left out. Think of it this way: once you have regained your beautiful or healthy body, you can finally do whatever you want. Since we have discussed the various kinds of fasting, maybe you can employ some of the methods to give time for your activities and food. But for now, finish your 30-day challenge. Increase the time you need until you gain a healthy lifestyle you have always needed if possible. Think of those declines and missed opportunities as an inspiration to look forward. You just have to tell them, "Not now."

How to Gain Unstoppable Self-Discipline

Furthermore, it is important to employ the best methods to have self-discipline in everything you do. To maintain the right hours for eating, fasting, and exercising, you are going to need to train your brain as a ticking clock. It needs to be wired up in the sense that you are given an alarm clock from within. In this way, you will not miss your meals, eat while you fast, deprive yourself of sleep, and be unable to maintain a regular physical exercise. Without further ado, here are some techniques to acquire unstoppable self-control.

Create a Mantra

Whenever you are unconfident about fasting, it is best to create an early morning mantra that starts with "I am." If you really aim to have a healthy and beautiful body, you can say, "I am strong enough to withstand any temptation today. In a few weeks, I will have the body I deserve to have." In cases where your self-discipline is challenged, you can close your eyes and say, "I am in control of my emotions and impulses. No person can command me of what I can do." Repeat these mantras ten times or more, whatever you see fit. But you still need to claim it and believe that you can do what you are talking about. Otherwise, your mantra will be all for nothing. Let it sink into your mind and heart. As it does, you are left with a burning fervor to carry over your plan.

Write in a Journal

A lot of people remain skeptic about writing all your thoughts and feelings in a journal. They say that it is a waste of time and energy because it does not do anything. On the contrary, journal writing is a very effective way to monitor your thoughts and feelings. It will be like giving yourself a pep talk whenever you feel like you are about to give up. Journal writing is a proven-and-tested method to pour down your feelings and feel good about yourself. Another fun fact is that this method actually helps in disciplining the mind. How do you ask? Writing entails focus and concentration. When you write in a journal, you are forcing your mind to dig deep within your level of subconscious and write everything you can think about in an orderly fashion. If you try this method, you can see a dramatic change in the way you organize your thoughts and control your emotions. Focus is the key, and this is one way you can train yourself to acquire it.

Practice Mindfulness in Everything

Mindfulness is defined as putting yourself in the moment and being aware of your environment. For instance, when you are aware of how, what, and why you eat, not only will you be able to enjoy a perfectly good meal but you will also practice control over your eating habits and methods. Think of it this way, when a person does not emancipate mindfulness during mealtime, you tend to stuff any food on the table in your mouth. You cannot pay attention to the leptin hormone signaling your body that it is already time to stop eating. You can observe that in people who watch the television while having a meal as they tend to be more obese than others who stay away from such distractions. That is because they merely focus on what they watch and not on their food intake.

Learn to Rest

People tend to be more emotional when they are restless. Imagine working graveyard shifts. Or, if you know someone who is totally restless, you know that they can be very irritable, angry, and dreadful. This is the reason why people easily give up. They feel tired in dealing with countless problems. When you are starting to feel this way, you should find a way to relax. When it is time for a break, get up from your chair and stretch or talk to your colleagues. Do not bring your work home if possible as well. Likewise, do not bring your family problems in the office. Learn to deal with things one at a time and try not to pressure yourself with everything else. When it is time to sleep at night, it is best to doze off for 7 to 8 hours to prepare yourself for a new day. Sleep and rest are known to rejuvenate the brain and body. They can put everything back in a state of balance along with all the chemicals and hormones. Finally, you are less stressed and less agitated when you wake up.

Share with Your Friends and Family

This is a very important method to increase your social support. When you have enough people to keep you motivated towards your growth and improvement, they will be more than happy to get you through your ordeals and trials. Ask them to help you deal with any temptation and not to mock you while you are trying to stick to a diet. Get their assistance to stay on the right track as well by lifting up your spirits when you feel down and encouraging you to become stronger. You will find yourself more motivated to continue on your venture and be more successful in reaching your goals.

Find New Hobbies

Hobbies are nice ways to get you distracted from food urges and frustrations. Boredom is one of your worst enemies when you are trying to fast. There are instances when people get too preoccupied on their thoughts and negative feelings when they feel bored. It's not that they are want to break their fasting, but they have nothing else to do. Thus, they are tempted to eat. We can observe several people who are inclined to eat whenever they get bored, so it is important to look for various things to get your mind off of the urge to eat, especially when you are with your friends and family.

Be Socially Involved

It is possible to look for organizations that support the cause of fasting in society. For this matter, you can learn a variety of methods on how you can venture into intermittent fasting more successfully. Plus, if you find people who will push you and motivate you towards fasting, you will be more inclined to eat only as scheduled. When you stay active in this group, you will realize that there are people with more problems than you. By talking to them, you can learn from their experiences and gather a hack or two from their wisdom.

Remove All Temptations

If you want to successfully accomplish your goal towards weight loss, get rid of anything that can tempt you into binge-eating. This includes emptying your refrigerator and cabinets of junk food and other unhealthy foods. Instead, fill it with tea, coffee, healthy beverages, and other liquids for rehydration. Whenever it is time to eat, avoid oily foods as much as you can and settle for vegetables and fruits for better effects.

Don't Wait for It to Feel Good

One of the many reasons why people give up on intermittent fasting is that they do not feel good about the method. Well, nothing really feels good in the beginning, especially when you are trying to change your former habits. After all, when people start to quit alcoholism and smoking, the start is always rocky. There will be withdrawal and perhaps even depression to deal with at times However, if you are committed to doing something positive for yourself, do not wait for it to feel good. It only gets better after a few days, weeks, or months. As we have been reiterating, do not let your emotions take control over your mind.

Learn to Schedule

When you have a poor sense of time, you better use an alarm to signal whether it is time to eat or not. Make a time frame for your workout routine as well. These things are important in slowly building a good habit that you can use in a lifetime.

Don't Be Too Hard on Yourself

At the beginning, it is inevitable to deal with failures and mistakes. But the mindset to successful fasting is not built overnight. You need to learn to forgive yourself and move forward. Otherwise, you will be stuck and feel depressed and anxious every bit of the way. You have all the time in the world to restart and retrace your steps. You should not feel too guilty when you fail on the first days of your intermittent-fasting sessions. Just promise yourself that whenever you slip up, you will never cease to get back up and keep trying.

Learn to Give Rewards

There is a concept in psychology called operant conditioning. Much like intermittent fasting, it is a method that has been around for centuries. Coined by B.F. Skinner in his early work between 1890 to 1930, operating conditioning ran supreme among many methods for behavior modification. It was based on Thorndike's Law of Effect, but with a little reinforcement. Skinner discovered this idea when he conducted an experiment on rats. He placed two levers in a box; when pulled, one would cause an electric shock, while the other would dispense pellets for the rats to eat. He found that the rodent avoided the electrocution lever and focused on pulling the one that would give them food. This concept can be applied to us humans in an effective fashion as well. When a person's mind is hardwired to think that a successful and good action constitutes a reward, you are likely to repeat the action again.

You can employ this method to train your mind and gain self-control while fasting intermittently, of course. You can reward yourself after a day of fasting efficiently by eating something that you love once it's time to break your fast. Better yet, you can give yourself something that you have always want to have after completing a whole week of successful fasting. When your brain starts to associate a positive thing with the practice, you are more likely to accomplish this goal one way or another despite the challenges it comes with.

Conclusion

Intermittent fasting is not just a hobby that people try for fun. This is a proven method that will allow you to start living healthier. Intermittent fasting was first introduced by the father of medicine, Hippocrates, and had been in the minds of people for generations. Many other proponents of science have also become advocates of this practice. From their studies, they have found that intermittent fasting is not only used for weight-loss purposes. The truth is, weight loss is only a bonus. Intermittent fasting was initially known to prevent cardiovascular disease, respiratory issues, diabetes, promotion of growth, and longevity. Imagine how healthy your body is going to be after finishing the 30-day intermittent fasting challenge.

Sadly, there are people who are not recommended to try fasting. They are the ones with depression, anorexia, and even a baby on the way. However, if you have the opportunity to grab this method and commit to it, you will not regret engaging every moment towards intermittent fasting. Sooner than later, you will find yourself in the brink of a healthy lifestyle, equipped with an alert mind and a strong body. Who said you cannot regain a sexy body after bearing three children? Who said you cannot have a healthy lifestyle when you reach 40 or 60 years old?

All it takes is a whole lot of commitment, confidence, and self-discipline. These three are the main components of a successful intermittent fasting routine. Without any of them, your journey is bound to cease and fail. It is not easy to lose weight - that is a fact. There will be people who might demean you, bully you even more, and doubt every bit of your spirit. So, you need to be ready to deal with them. Never listen to naysayers and negative thinkers; instead, surround yourself with individuals who will love, accept, and support you in every venture that you choose. Your real friends and family will be happy to hear that you are doing something to improve yourself. The rest might undermine you because of it, but they should not matter anyway. As we have said earlier, you are not doing this for them. In fact, you are doing it for yourself. Think of the long-term effects of your intermittent fasting. Soon, you will be able to wear that sexy dress in the store and flaunt your body that has become healthy both inside and out.

I admire people with such grit and to change their bad habits wholeheartedly. They are willing to sacrifice their old hobbies for the betterment of their heart, mind, and soul. If you have read this book from cover to cover, it means that you have taken the first step towards having a successful life, and I want to congratulate you for it. It is not easy to put in so much effort in a book when you can just do other things. I hope that I have motivated you to become a stronger, fuller, and healthier woman. Always remember that you are beautiful. You are unique. You have spectacular talents. Let this book be a beacon towards a healthy mind and body. This way, you can imagine being on the front porch of your home, getting ready for work or school, and feeling confident as ever. You are now looking forward to meeting other people because you know all the positive changes that you have undergone internally are now visible externally. You no longer have to suffer the endless name-calling from ill-meaning people. You no longer have to endure the stares at restaurants, buses, and trains. You are now a changed woman, holistically speaking. Not only have you developed a healthy lifestyle but an amazing mindset as well. That is what intermittent fasting can do to you.

Bibliography

Australian Professional Skills Institute (2016). 7 time management tips for students. Retrieved from https://www.apsi.edu.au/7-time-management-tips-students/

Barnosky, A., Hoddy, K., Unterman, T., & Varady, K. (2014). Intermittent fasting vs daily calorie restriction for type 2 diabetes prevention: a review of human findings. Retrieved from https://www.translationalres.com/article/S1931-5244(14)00200-X/abstract

Bilich, K. (n.d.). 10 benefits of physical activity. Retrieved from https://www.parents.com/fun/sports/exercise/10-benefits-of-physical-activity/

Brazier, Y. (2018). Measuring BMI for adults, children, and teens. Retrieved from https://www.medicalnewstoday.com/articles/323622.php

Campbell-Avenell, Z. (2016). 49 ways to say no to anyone (when you don't want to be a jerk). Retrieved from https://www.careerfaqs.com.au/news/news-and-views/how-to-say-no-to-anyone

Charkalis, D. (2018). 13 dos and don'ts of intermittent fasting. Retrieved from https://www.livestrong.com/slideshow/1008373-master-fast-dos-donts/?slide=1

Cole, W. (n.d.). Intermittent fasting: A complete guide to benefits, diet plans & meals. Retrieved from https://www.mindbodygreen.com/articles/intermittent-fasting-diet-plan-how-to-schedule-meals

Crosta, P. (2017). Everything you need to know about cellulite. Retrieved from https://www.medicalnewstoday.com/articles/149465.php

Donelly, C. (n.d.). The do's and don'ts of intermittent fasting [Slideshow]. Retrieved from https://www.sharecare.com/health/diet-nutrition/slideshow/the-dos-and-donts-intermittent-fasting#slide-1

Fielding, S. (2019). Wondering why your beer belly is hard? Here are 5 possible causes. A rock-hard stomach isn't always a good thing. Retrieved from https://www.menshealth.com/weight-loss/a19543924/abs-diet-hard-belly-fat/

Foundation Education (2016). 5 essential self-management skills. Retrieved from https://www.foundationeducation.edu.au/articles/2016/10/5-self-management-skills-you-need-to-win-at-life

Fung, J. (n.d.). Fasting – A History Part I. Retrieved from https://idmprogram.com/fasting-a-history-part-i/

Gould, H. (2019). This explains so much: Turns Out we all have 4 different types of fat. Retrieved from https://www.byrdie.com/how-to-lose-fat

Gunnars, K. (2017). What is intermittent fasting? Explained in human terms. Retrieved from https://www.healthline.com/nutrition/what-is-intermittent-fasting

Greenlaw, P. & Greenlaw D. (2016). The history of dieting and weight loss: It started 2,300 years ago with the Greeks. Retrieved from https://www.christianpost.com/news/the-history-of-dieting-and-weight-loss-it-started-2300-years-ago-with-the-greeks.html

Harris, S. (2018). What happens if you fast for a day? Retrieved from https://www.medicalnewstoday.com/articles/322065.php

Harvard Health Publishing. (2017). Not so fast: Pros and cons of the newest diet trend. Retrieved from https://www.health.harvard.edu/heart-health/not-so-fast-pros-and-cons-of-the-newest-diet-trend

Holmes, P. (2010). The different types of fast. Retrieved from https://www.crosswalk.com/faith/women/the-different-types-of-fasts-11626299.html

Institute of Medicine (US) Subcommittee on Military Weight Management. (2004). Weight management: State of the science and opportunities for military programs. Washington D.C: National Academies Press. Retrieved from https://www.ncbi.nlm.nih.gov/books/NBK221834/

Jarreau, P. (2018). Your menstrual cycle on intermittent fasting. Retrieved from https://lifeapps.io/fasting/your-menstrual-cycle-on-intermittent-fasting/

Koman, T. (2018). 10 celebrities who swear by intermittent fasting. Retrieved from https://www.delish.com/food/g22617665/celebrities-intermittent-fasting/

Land, S. (2018). 15 different types of intermittent fasting and their benefits. Retrieved from https://siimland.com/15-different-types-of-intermittent-fasting-and-their-benefits/

Lefave, S. (2018). 8 major mistakes people make when intermittent fasting. Retrieved from https://whatsgood.vitaminshoppe.com/intermittent-fasting-mistakes/

Lewis, D. (2013). Explainer: Why do women menstruate? Retrieved from http://theconversation.com/explainer-why-do-women-menstruate-13744

Link, R. (2018). 8 health benefits of fasting, backed by science. Retrieved from https://www.healthline.com/nutrition/fasting-benefits

Lizzy Loves Food. (2019). My 30 days on intermittent fasting results. Retrieved from https://lizzylovesfood.com/30-day-intermittent-fasting-results/

Lowery, M. (2017). Top 5 intermittent fasting mistakes. Retrieved from https://2mealday.com/article/top-5-intermittent-fasting-mistakes/

Maternity Comfort Solutions. (2018). 7 intermittent fasting hacks to lose the baby weight. Retrieved from https://maternitycomfortsolutions.com/7-intermittent-fasting-hacks-for-losing-the-baby-weight/

McLeod, S. (2018). Skinner – Operant conditioning. Retrieved from https://www.simplypsychology.org/operant-conditioning.html

Mercola. J. (2013). Should you eat before exercise? Retrieved from https://fitness.mercola.com/sites/fitness/archive/2013/09/13/eating-before-exercise.aspx

National Eating Disorders Association. (n.d.). Anorexia nervosa. Retrieved from https://www.nationaleatingdisorders.org/learn/by-eating-disorder/anorexia

Nursing Times. (2009). Malnutrition. Retrieved from https://www.nursingtimes.net/malnutrition/5001811.article

Pedre, V. (n.d.). Intermittent fasting can be dangerous for some people. Here's exactly what you need to know. Retrieved from https://www.mindbodygreen.com/0-29932/intermittent-fasting-can-be-dangerous-for-some-people-heres-exactly-what-you-need-to-know.html

Pique. (n.d.). What to drink while intermittent fasting. Retrieved from https://blog.piquetea.com/what-to-drink-while-intermittent-fasting/

Polevoi, L. (n.d.). 8 tips for effective time management. Retrieved from https://quickbooks.intuit.com/r/employees/8-tips-for-effective-time-management/

PTI. (2018). Here's why women gain weight after pregnancy. Retrieved from https://www.deccanchronicle.com/lifestyle/health-and-wellbeing/100718/heres-why-women-gain-weight-after-pregnancy.html

Rampton, J. (2018). Manipulate time with these powerful 20 time management tips. Retrieved on https://www.forbes.com/sites/johnrampton/2018/05/01/manipulate-time-with-these-powerful-20-time-management-tips/#733967a857ab

Randone, A. (2018). What happens when you get your period during Ramadan. Retrieved from https://www.teenvogue.com/story/what-happens-when-you-get-your-period-during-ramadan

Rettner, R. (2016). The 4 types of exercise you need to be healthy. Retrieved from https://www.livescience.com/55317-exercise-types.html

Romm, A. (n.d.). 7 steps to get over food cravings & gain control of your life. Retrieved from https://www.mindbodygreen.com/0-13876/7-steps-to-get-over-food-cravings-gain-control-of-your-life.html

Science Daily. (n.d.). Adipose tissue. Retrieved from https://www.sciencedaily.com/terms/adipose_tissue.htm

Skills You Need. (n.d.). Dealing with stress - Ten tips. Retrieved from https://www.skillsyouneed.com/ps/stress-tips.html

Smith, L. & Lunders, K. (n.d.). 20 weight loss motivation quotes that will empower you to keep going. Retrieved from https://www.womansday.com/health-fitness/womens-health/g3209/best-weight-loss-motivation/

Spritzler, F. (2017). 16 foods to eat on a ketogenic diet. Retrieved from https://www.healthline.com/nutrition/ketogenic-diet-foods

Steve. (n.d.). How to build your own workout routine. Retrieved from https://www.nerdfitness.com/blog/how-to-build-your-own-workout-routine/

Streit, L. (2018). Malnutrition: Definition, symptoms, and treatment. Retrieved from https://www.healthline.com/nutrition/malnutrition

Taylor, M. (2018). 9 things you must do to lose weight over 40, according to experts. Retrieved from https://www.prevention.com/weight-loss/a20465042/lose-weight-over-40/

Thompson, C. (n.d.). 7 types of fast. Retrieved from https://www.livestrong.com/article/520268-7-types-of-fasts/

West, H. (2019). How to fast safely: 10 helpful tips. Retrieved from https://www.healthline.com/nutrition/how-to-fast

Whiteman, H. (2015). Fasting: health benefits and risks. Retrieved from https://www.medicalnewstoday.com/articles/295914.php

World Health Organization. (2018). Obesity and overweight. Retrieved from https://www.who.int/news-room/fact-sheets/detail/obesity-and-overweight